LOVE YOUR ASIAN BODY

LOVE YOUR ASIAN BODY

AIDS ACTIVISM IN LOS ANGELES

ERIC C. WAT

UNIVERSITY OF WASHINGTON PRESS | *Seattle*

Design by Katrina Noble
Composed in Hoftype Cala, typeface designed by Dieter Hofrichter

25   24   23   22   21   5   4   3   2   1

Printed and bound in the United States of America

UNIVERSITY OF WASHINGTON PRESS
uwapress.uw.edu

LIBRARY OF CONGRESS CATALOGING-IN-PUBLICATION DATA ON FILE
Names: Wat, Eric C., 1970– author.
Title: Love your Asian body : AIDS activism in Los Angeles / Eric C. Wat.
Description: Seattle : University of Washington Press, [2021] |
    Includes bibliographical references and index.
Identifiers: LCCN 2021003569 (print) | LCCN 2021003570 (ebook) |
    ISBN 9780295749327 (hardcover) | ISBN 9780295749334 (paperback) |
    ISBN 9780295749341 (ebook)
Subjects: LCSH: Asian Pacific AIDS Intervention Team—History. | AIDS
    activists—California—Los Angeles—Interviews. | AIDS (Disease)—
    Social aspects—California—Los Angeles. | HIV infections—Social aspects—
    California—Los Angeles. | Asian Americans—Diseases. | Pacific Islander
    Americans—Diseases. | Asian American gays—California—Los Angeles—
    Social conditions. | Pacific Islander American gays—California—
    Los Angeles—Social conditions.
Classification: LCC RA643.84.C2 W38 2021 (print) | LCC RA643.84.C2 (ebook) |
    DDC 362.19697/9200979494—dc23
LC record available at https://lccn.loc.gov/2021003569
LC ebook record available at https://lccn.loc.gov/2021003570

The paper used in this publication is acid free and meets the minimum requirements of American National Standard for Information Sciences—Permanence of Paper for Printed Library Materials, ANSI Z39.48-1984.∞

For James E. Sakakura (1958–1996)

CONTENTS

ACKNOWLEDGMENTS

I am indebted to the following brave souls who entrusted me with their life stories: Noel Alumit, Robert Berger, Tom Callahan, Oscar de la O, Ghalib Shiraz Dhalla, J Craig Fong, Heng Lam Foong, Terry Gock, Dean Goishi, Shawn Griffin, Lisa Hasegawa, Herbert K. Hatanaka, Alice Y. Hom, JJ Joo, Karen Kimura Joo, Sally Jue, Naomi Kageyama, Pauline Kamiyama, Dredge Kang, Unhei Kang, Keith Kasai, Juan Lombard, Napoleon Lustre, Gil Mangaoang, Tracy Nako, Ric Parish, Stephano Park, Eric E. Reyes, Mark Sakakura, Patricia Sakakura, Margaret Endo Shimada, Joël Barraquiel Tan, Diep Tran, Phill Wilson, Connie Wong, and an anonymous narrator. I'm also thankful to Jeff Kim, Nobuko Miyamoto, Diane Ujiiye for supplying crucial information about this history. I regret that I couldn't fit all their stories in this book. You can find more stories on my author's website, www.ericwatbooks.com.

The book is the culmination of a research project conducted in collaboration with the Asian Pacific AIDS Intervention Team. Thank you to APAIT director Jury Candelario and his team, especially Abigail Proff, Jimmy Sianipar, and Daniel Nguyen, for their help since the beginning, when the idea was but a germ. I am also grateful to the ONE Archives Foundation, whose support for the archival research for this project was so valuable. Loni Shibuyama at ONE was especially helpful in guiding me through its AIDS History Project collection. We also received funding from California Humanities to produce the podcast *Sex Positive*, based on these interviews, and to organize a series of community dialogues with activists, artists, and survivors of the epidemic. Hannah Harris

Green is the producer of the podcast, and Irene Suico Soriano co-curated one of the community dialogues with me. The podcast is available at http://apaitonline.org/sexpositive/.

In 2017, with help from APAIT staff, we launched a crowdfunding campaign to raise money for research expenses. In just six weeks, we raised over $7,000 from more than a hundred donors. The names of these early supporters are listed on my author's website, www.ericwatbooks.com.

The publication process was not as arduous as I had feared. For that, I have the following angels to thank: Crystal Baik, Tammy Ho, Linda España Maram, Anthony Ocampo, and Peter Park offered insights for the query process. At the University of Washington Press, my editors Larin R. McLaughlin and Mike Baccam and staff member Jason Alley shepherded the manuscript with their gentle and nurturing hands. Art director Katrina Noble designed the cover image that illustrated perfectly the joyousness that the activists cultivated against all odds, even during the grimmest years of the epidemic. The spot-on copyediting by Richard Feit made my words tighter and cleaner, and his collaborative spirit made the revision process one that I looked forward to. There were so many other resources from the University of Washington Press that I am not able to list them all here; thankfully, project editor Joeth Zucco managed the production process to make sure all the magic happened at the right time.

Finally, before I wrote the first word for this book, I had been agonizing over the tone that I would use to do justice to these stories. When I brought up this dilemma to my therapist, Lance Tango, he asked me, "What do you think the tone of your life is?" After I settled down from such a heavy question, we decided that in our sessions, I'd always worked on honing empathy, in my relationships with others and with myself. "Why try to be someone different when you write?" asked Lance. With that advice, I typed the first word the next day, and I didn't stop until I was done. I hope empathy is what the narrators and readers can discern from these pages.

LOVE YOUR ASIAN BODY

Introduction

AIDS ISN'T JUST A DISEASE; IT'S ALSO A MOVEMENT. AT THE epidemic's onset in the 1980s, mystery and misinformation surrounded the disease that was yet to be named. By the middle of that decade, a group of queer Asian American men and women in Los Angeles came together and provided support for those in their community who were sick and dying. They became caregivers, nurses, social workers, researchers, and advocates for Asian Americans living with HIV. They built a community infrastructure, without which many more people would have contracted the virus and died.

I was one of those people the movement saved. I had immigrated to the US in the summer of 1982, just before I turned twelve. I was beginning to wrestle with my attraction to men, a tortuous process made only more so by the specter of AIDS. An AIDS diagnosis in those days was a death sentence. AIDS paranoia struck Asian American gay men in different ways. Some became infected because no one told them the risks and how to circumvent them. Among this group, recent immigrants with limited English proficiency were the hardest to reach. Or they were rendered so invisible by the racism in the gay community or trapped by their community's homophobia that they would assume the risks in exchange for a chance encounter of recognition and pleasure.

With access to information and resources, I was privileged. By the time I went to college in late 1980s, I had found a community of Asian American queers radicalized by AIDS and other political struggles. Luckily for me, this coincided with the vibrant AIDS organizing in the Asian American community in Los Angeles. The Asian American activists I profile in this book didn't save me only by teaching me how to protect myself from the virus. They saved me through their work fashioning

3

a new queer Asian American identity that allowed for fuller and more integrated racial, sexual, and political expressions for a new generation. Without a blueprint, these activists often had to be creative and agitational. Their experimentation had its share of mistakes, sometimes complicated by their own grief from the deaths around them. Yet this movement was unique in at least three aspects.

First, the Asian American AIDS activists had a sweeping vision that was not limited to AIDS. Rather, they saw AIDS as a nexus from which to address broader systemic issues. This vision led to the founding of the Asian Pacific AIDS Intervention Team (APAIT) in 1992 and continued to inform how they coalesced with other communities of color, such as the Gay Men of Color Consortium, at a time when Los Angeles was known for its interracial tensions.

Second, the activists advocated on behalf of the most stigmatized populations in their community, namely people living with HIV. In an age of political expediency, when strategists picked the lowest hanging fruit (and often stopped there), these activists chose the hardest fight and refused to back down from difficult conversations with people who didn't want to engage them, often in immigrant communities that were supposedly averse to discussing (gay) sex. They understood that in order to encourage at-risk people in immigrant communities to seek help, they first must change the social norms about sexuality in these communities. By pushing difficult conversations, the activists shed light on and humanized LGBTQ Asian Americans, regardless of their HIV status, and they sounded a clarion call to my generation to action. Like a tide lifting all boats, the AIDS movement was a potent form of community building in Los Angeles in the 1990s.

In discussing the challenges of AIDS outreach and education in immigrant communities, I caution readers not to infer that Asians (or Asian cultures) are more homophobic than mainstream US society. There are certain factors that make many Asian cultures *differently* homophobic. The emphases on filial responsibility, harmony, and communal needs over individual ones, values that otherwise are protective factors against a racist society, can often make it hard for Asian Americans to live openly as LGBTQ people. In my previous book, *The Making of a Gay Asian Community*, a narrator, an immigrant from Malaysia, fed with romantic ideals about American progressivism, was shocked to find how blatantly discriminatory and even violent White Americans were toward LGBTQ people, whereas in his homeland, he was able to carry out relationships with other men as long as he fulfilled his duties as a son and did not flaunt his same-sex attraction. (His gender and class status in Malaysia also protected him from outright recriminations.) The vibrancy of the LGBTQ movement in the US, often used as an exhibit for Western enlightenment about sexuality, was a resistance against state-sanctioned violence against the LGBTQ community. As at least one narrator in this book attests, much of the homophobia they encountered in the Asian American community came from Christianity, a vestige of Western colonization in Asia. Homophobia cannot be dissected so cleanly and measured with objectivity and precision. The epidemic made LGBTQ people even more of a pariah in any community, and to combat homophobia in diverse communities required unique expertise and credibility—what the nonprofit sector came to call "cultural competence." Asian American AIDS advocates often used this cultural explanation to their advantage when arguing for funding equity, but the nuances could get lost with people who were stuck in the mythology of the antiquated and changeless East.

Finally, the Asian American AIDS activists centered pleasure in the movement. In reinforcing the sexual agency of LGBTQ Asian Americans, they made sex and pleasure an integral part of community organizing. Raunchy sex education wasn't just an advertising stunt. It reinforced a sex-positive ideology that anyone—whether they preferred their sex "vanilla" or "kinky," whether they were in a traditional or polyamorous relationship—deserved to have access to good health care and to thrive in a community. Their embrace of deviance was no small feat, considering how the epidemic had walked back much of the promise of freedom in gender and sexual expressions from a previous generation. In so doing, they reclaimed queer sex and modeled inclusiveness of nonconformity as notions of gender and sexuality continue to evolve to this day.

The stories of these AIDS activists and survivors collected in this volume took place primarily in Los Angeles between the mid-1980s and mid-1990s. Race and class segregate Los Angeles, even after redlining and racial covenants were outlawed. The segregation is further reinforced by the freeways; as the saying goes, "Nobody walks in LA." You can drive, day in and day out, through a neighborhood and yet never come to know it. I have often told transplants from other cities, "It's easy to hate LA because you actually have to work at loving it."

A center of increasingly globalized economy in the Pacific Rim, LA is the site of multiple and continuous waves of migration from Asia, which became more intensified with the passage of the Immigration and Nationality Act in 1965 and the US defeat in its wars in Southeast Asia in the 1970s. Ethnic enclaves are often the markers of the rich diversity within the Asian American community. In LA, going from north to south, you have Thai Town in Hollywood; Chinatown, Historic Filipinotown (Hi-Fi), Little Tokyo, Koreatown, and Little Bangladesh in Central LA (the boundaries of the latter two overlap, not without controversy); Little India in Artesia; and Cambodia Town in Long Beach. Ethnic enclaves are just the tip of a very deceptive iceberg. Suburbanization has diluted the concentration of many of these enclaves. More and more Asian American families live in municipalities in the San Gabriel Valley, the San Fernando Valley, South Bay, Long Beach, and even the Westside, which has a history of exclusion of people of color. In some cities, particularly in the San Gabriel Valley and South Bay, Asian Americans constitute significant pluralities or even majorities.

The ability to move out of traditional ethnic enclaves has meant some degree of assimilation to and economic success in mainstream US society. Many ethnic enclaves are no longer the launching pads for recent immigrants they once were, even when the flagship community organizations that serve specific ethnic groups still headquarter there.

The decentralization of the Asian American community—not to mention its cultural and linguistic diversity—presented a challenge for early AIDS activists. For every message to any ethnic community, they had to consider not only the words themselves, but also their connotation, tone, and resonance. Then they had to find the right partners to help get the word out. For immigrants most at risk, messengers in their community, otherwise trusted for most issues, might be the last people from which they would seek help and advice about HIV. A one-size-fits-all approach often came up short because many Asian immigrants didn't have a meaningful connection to a pan-ethnic identity. AIDS activists had to be creative, resourceful, strategic, and persistent in order to be equitable and inclusive of all communities (though sometimes failing at it). But this diversity, despite its many challenges, should be seen for its richness. In the 1990s, there was an explosion of LGBTQ Asian American groups in LA, mostly along ethnic lines. These organizations were strategic sites for AIDS organizing, and in turn, AIDS funding drove their growth during that decade and built their leadership. These ethnic-specific organizations provided rare and vital spaces for at-risk immigrants to find community and support.

Between 2017 and 2019, I interviewed thirty-six people for this book. Their stories are interwoven in eighteen chapters.

The AIDS epidemic did not arise out of a vacuum. Chapter 1 ("Brand New World") delves into the tensions between conservative mores and radical possibilities that played out in the decade before the epidemic, embodied in the relationship between AIDS activist/survivor Gil Mangaoang and Juan Lombard. Chapter 2 ("Universal Precautions") explores AIDS paranoia in the early years of the epidemic, even among health professionals and gay men. The resulting discrimination against people with AIDS was a driving force behind the activism of many, including social worker Sally Jue.

The next three chapters discuss the beginning of the community's effort to build an infrastructure to fight the epidemic. For different reasons, as late as the mid-1980s, many gay Asian men were reluctant to take on AIDS as a collective struggle. Chapter 3 ("A Rumor of Plague") tells the story of how a small group of members within the insular Asian/Pacific Lesbians and Gays (A/PLG), including Dean Goishi, formed a committee called the AIDS Intervention Team (AIT) in 1987, despite the indifference of the organization's leadership. The movement received a boost in 1991, when many young people were galvanized by then governor Pete Wilson's veto of a bill that would prohibit discrimination against LGBTQ people. Chapter 4 ("Fuck That") discusses how a new generation of queer Asian American activists, like Joël Barraquiel Tan and Ric Parish, focused on AIDS to mobilize their community. They eventually joined with the older activists at AIT. The influx of these younger and more radical activists led to its split from A/PLG and the founding of the Asian Pacific AIDS Intervention Team (APAIT) in 1992. The story of this secession is told in Chapter 5 ("Exit Strategies").

Chapters 6 to 13 chart the growth of APAIT from a scrappy group of grassroots activists to one of the more formidable forces in the AIDS service landscape through the mid-1990s. Early on, APAIT strategically allied with AIDS organizations in other communities of color to advocate for more equitable funding for non-White populations. Chapter 6 ("School of Fish") recounts how APAIT was able to secure more funding from the county as part of the Gay Men of Color Consortium. Their success allowed them to build out their team. Chapter 7 ("The Young and the Fearless") tells the stories of early APAIT staff, who were mostly hired to conduct outreach and education. Chapter 8 ("Filthy, Dirty Ads") describes APAIT's first social marketing campaign in 1992, which challenged the racial discourse in the local gay and lesbian community. Its success led to later social marketing campaigns, which are detailed in Chapter 9 ("Do Your Job. Piss Somebody Off."). Through these campaigns, APAIT began to speak to Asian immigrant communities about the taboo subjects of AIDS and sexuality.

APAIT later received funding to provide services directly to Asian Americans living with HIV, including case management and a drop-in center that created social opportunities for HIV-positive clients. These programs are described in Chapter 10 ("Interpreters of Maladies"). This work proved their cultural and linguistic competence in serving the diverse Asian American community and led to funding for more specialized direct services, including treatment advocacy and mental health counseling. Chapter 11 ("We Want a New Drug") describes the uneasy relationship between drug companies and AIDS activists and profiles Ric Parish, who pioneered treatment advocacy at the organization. Chapter 12 ("That Shrinking Window of Reconciliation") tells the stories of Keith Kasai (APAIT volunteer and client) and Margaret Endo Shimada (mental health counselor) and how counseling contributes to more positive perceptions in the Asian American community not only of HIV-positive individuals, but also of LGBTQ people in general. The mid-1990s witnessed an explosion of ethnic-specific LGBTQ organizations in the Asian American community. Chapter 13 ("What AIDS Animated") reveals the symbiotic relationship between APAIT and these queer organizations, specifically in Korean, South Asian, and Vietnamese women's communities.

No story about the AIDS movement can be complete without discussion about love and grief. AIDS challenged the ways that gay men could relate to one another romantically and sexually. Chapter 14 ("The Dating Pool") talks about the blurred boundaries between staff and community when finding love and romance. The close-knit relationships made any AIDS-related death that much more traumatic. Chapter 15 ("Good Grief") describes the different ways that APAIT staff processed their grief. The death that caused the biggest trauma at that time was that of beloved APAIT staff member James Sakakura. Chapter 16 ("This Darkness Is Not Your Life") recounts James's life and death through his surviving mother, Patricia, and eldest brother, Mark, including James's struggles with addiction and his loves and friendships in the movement.

The Asian American AIDS movement in LA was not always one big happy family. The AIDS movement was not immune to sexism. Chapter 17 ("Not to be Dicked Around") describes the many contributions of Asian American women to the movement, despite many examples of male chauvinism. The most egregious was a fundraiser in 1993 on the eve of a national AIDS conference hosted by APAIT, where performers enacted a comedic sketch that made light of domestic violence. The fallout caused a rift not only within the local community, but also between APAIT and activists in other cities. Finally, Chapter 18 ("Downright Respectable") explains how APAIT became a victim of its own success in the mid-1990s. Its growth in funding and services was often achieved at the expense of the grassroots activism that birthed the organization. Medical advancement also shifted the focus from broader cultural change to individualized treatment. The radical activism from the early years began to diminish. This last chapter also offers examples of how the local Asian American AIDS movement has attempted to stay relevant in the new millennium.

In our interviews, almost all the narrators used the term Asian and Pacific Islander or API to describe their community. Throughout the 1980s and 1990s, there was an attempt by the Asian American community to be in alliance with Pacific Islanders, as reflected by the inclusion of the word *Pacific* in the names of many local and national pan-ethnic organizations. This was often reinforced by government funding categories that lumped the two groups together. This aspiration has seldom panned out. The cultures and experiences of Pacific Islanders in the US are vastly different from those of Asians. In my interviews with the AIDS activists, their narratives, while focusing on such broad topics as the model-minority myth, for example, or outreach in immigrant communities, did not include Pacific Islander meaningfully. Therefore, I use the term *Asian American* in this book to describe this movement history, except in direct quotations by the narrators.

There is some urgency in telling these stories now. We've already lost too many to AIDS over the years, and those who have survived are getting older and frailer. This book is my love letter to both the city and the people who were part of this AIDS movement in the Asian American community, not only those I've interviewed for this book, but the many more with whom I was unable to speak.

In July 2017, I flew across the country to interview my first narrator, Dean Goishi, APAIT cofounder and founding director, at his home in Florida, where he is now retired. He and his partner picked me up at the airport. On the ride home, Dean, who was well into his seventies, turned to me and said, "I'm afraid you've wasted a trip. I don't think I remember that much." But when we adjourned to their sunroom at 9:30 the next morning after breakfast and Dean pulled out a pack of Japanese rice crackers from the tidy compartment of his walker and settled in next to me, the memories came in a stream, story after story after story. An hour and a half later, I asked if he needed a break. He said we could keep going. Shortly after 1 p.m., almost four hours after we began, I told him *I* needed a break.

We think we forget. But there is another relationship we have with memories between remembering and forgetting. AIDS lives there for most of us. Maybe we could tell the story of AIDS only when we could do it collectively.

But this is not just an exercise in nostalgia. I have written this book also for younger generations of activists. Political realities will evolve; strategies will become outdated. But the creative imagination to always seek a better alternative, the youthful courage to experiment, and the joy to fight for what is right remain constants in any social movement. A heteronormative society severs queer people from our past and leaves us without any tradition, isolated and ahistorical. With this book, I aim to say to younger queer Asian Americans, *You are not alone. You've come from a powerful lineage.*

CHAPTER 1

Brand New World

THE FIRST FIVE CASES OF AIDS IN THE US WERE DETECTED IN young gay White men in Los Angeles in 1981. AIDS activists of color believed that if the *Morbidity and Mortality Weekly Report* by the Centers for Disease Control and Prevention had gone deeper than these first five, they would have found many more people of color afflicted. This was one of the first lessons of the epidemic. Our public health priorities were based on what got reported to the government, and what got reported to the government reflected who had access to our health care system and who didn't.

In part due to this misperception of those whom the disease afflicted, the response to the AIDS crisis in the Asian American community in LA didn't begin until 1987, when a handful of members in Asian/Pacific Lesbians and Gays (A/PLG) formed a committee called the AIDS Intervention Team. Their small-scale efforts were initially directed internally, at their members only. By 1991, with additional funding, this committee broke away from its parent organization and became the Asian Pacific AIDS Intervention Team (APAIT), which is still thriving today. In 1994, Eric Reyes, while a management consultant for APAIT, testified at the Los Angeles County HIV Commission that "the API [Asian/Pacific Islander] community is a keg of dynamite ready to explode. . . . The consensus is that APIs are about five years behind in HIV education/prevention efforts compared to the gay White male community."

As tardy as the Asian American response might have been, it didn't materialize out of thin air. Rather, it was built on years of political experience and connections of community leaders. Take Gil Mangaoang, for instance. In the 1990s, Gil would become first a client at APAIT and then one of its managers on staff. Around the time of the Stonewall Rebellion, however, Gil, then in his early twenties, was just discovering his attraction to men. "My first sexual experience with a man was when I was in the Air Force," Gil recounted. "He picked me up at the Janis Joplin concert [laughs] in Centennial Park. Ever since then, I got hooked." Raised by a father who was a fundamentalist Pentecostal minister—"We're bible-thumpers to the core"—Gil continued to date women while "playing around with men on the side."

After he was discharged from the Air Force in 1970, Gil went to school at City College of San Francisco, where his racial identity was radicalized. In the shadow of the Third World Liberation Front student strike for ethnic studies at San Francisco State University just the year before, Gil joined with other Filipino American students and learned about the history of Filipinos in the US. They demanded courses on Philippine history and Tagalog language and advocated for racial parity in faculty hiring. His activism attracted the attention of leftists in the local Filipino American community. In 1971 he was invited to join the Kalayaan Collective, which was influenced by the teachings of Third World communists like Mao Tse-Tung and José Maria (Joma) Sison. Through Kalayaan, Gil fought on the side of retired Filipino farmworkers (*manongs*) who were being evicted from the International Hotel, and he organized local efforts in support of overseas resistance to the regime of Ferdinand Marcos, the Philippine dictator who rose to power with US backing.

When the Kalayaan Collective folded in 1972, Gil seamlessly moved onto another leftist group called Katipunan ng mga Demokratikong Pilipino (KDP). Among other activities, KDP organized national conventions where progressive Filipino activists would meet and network. It was at the second People's Far West Convention in 1972 in Stockton where he "got together" with Annie, who would shortly become his fiancée. Like a power couple, Annie and Gil moved up the leadership ladder at KDP in lockstep.

Gil quickly moved in with Annie, who was living with her mother on Polk Street in San Francisco. This proved to be the "downfall" in their relationship. "Annie's mother had this nice little black dog named Gigi," he explained. "Of course, dogs need to be walked. I would volunteer to walk Gigi. And Gigi needed to be walked on Polk Street." Gil told this story with a mischievous grin. Since the 1950s, Polk Gulch had been the main gay neighborhood in San Francisco, until the bars and their patrons started migrating to the gentrifying Castro in the late 1970s. During these dog walks, Gil would take every opportunity to meet men and satisfy his sexual desire, which couldn't be sated with his relationship with Annie.

Three years into the relationship, Gil decided he couldn't lie to Annie anymore. He came clean and told her that she "deserved to have a full life." Annie told him the same thing, and the two broke up. Though it seemed amicable at first, their continued activism in KDP made things awkward. It didn't help that other people took sides, mostly Annie's. Gil said they believed he "was leaving this poor woman," whom he had "misled." Many of the leftist organizations at the time toed the line, drawn by their overseas communist influences, that homosexuality was a perverted byproduct of capitalism, which, like prostitution or child abuse, would evaporate easily in a classless society. Gil's sexuality was seen not only as a personal betrayal to Annie, but also a political betrayal to the larger group. Despite having strong female (and ironically, lesbian) leadership, KDP was not immune to occasional charges of "male chauvinism." With the perceived slights against his former lover, Gil thought he was made a convenient scapegoat. He was forced to sit in discussion after discussion to "struggle with his male chauvinism"—a less severe version of reeducation camps in the new communist countries abroad, where any members who didn't fit the revolutionary model were pressured to confess and atone for their reactionary sins.

In rebellion to such degrading experiences, Gil flaunted his sexual identity scandalously. In an autobiographical essay, he wrote:

> I enjoyed the game of flirting with the straight political guys. In fact, there was a period of time when I just came out, that I went out of my way to be outrageous in how I expressed my declaration about being 'gay and proud.' Most of the time it just meant wearing an earring and lots of body jewelry, I felt that the shock value of outrageous behavior was a positive way of asserting my sexual identity. These youthful

actions were a passive-aggressive way of seeking recognition without the responsibility of having to justify my actions.[1]

In the same essay, Gil described a meeting at a KDP member's house where he and a comrade went into one of the bedrooms to have sex before the meeting began, making noises loud enough for others to hear.

As an out gay man, Gil began to envision relationships with other men, beyond the fleeting encounters on Polk Street or underhanded flirting. Gil looked to other gay leftist organizations in San Francisco, including the June 28th Union, whose name referred to the date of the Stonewall Rebellion. The first man he fell in love with was Ferd Eggan, a cofounder of ACT UP Chicago who later served as the AIDS coordinator for LA from 1993 to 2001. In the 1970s, Eggan explored the confluences of the Black Power, anti-war, and gay liberation movements. This took him to different cities to network with other activists, and the relationship between Gil and Ferd never really took hold.

Though he was "heartbroken" by this first gay romance, Gil started dating Jerry Michael Kraus, another young leader in the June 28th Union. "The KDP was really one of the more premier left organizations that people looked up to because of its sophistication," Gil explained. "Michael knew I was a member. He was very intrigued politically to understand our analytical processes, our ideological foundations and tenets. We had that intimate personal, sexual, and political relationship." As intense as the relationship was, it lasted only about three months.

One morning in July 1976, Gil was at work in his office in Oakland after another long meeting the previous night. "All political meetings last forever. It's coffee, coke, and cigarettes. Coca-Cola, mind you, not coke [cocaine]," Gil quipped. Eggan was calling him at work and leaving messages, like he had been for the past three days since the two had last seen one another. Gil had been ignoring Eggan's calls because he was exhausted. In Eggan's last message that day, he said he would come to Gil's office to talk to him. Gil relented. When they were alone, Eggan related the tragic news of Michael's being hit by a car as he was crossing 19th Street in the Dolores Mission District, almost home from yet another political meeting.

Gil was incredulous. He had just seen Michael at the anti-bicentennial demonstration, where a coalition of leftist organizations paraded down

Market Street. He held one end of a banner, and Gil the other. Gil asked Eggan if he could see Michael's body.

"You're too late," Eggan said. "That's why I've been trying to call you." Michael's body had already been shipped back to his family in New Jersey.

Gil was inconsolable. Worse, he couldn't share his grief with his families, biological or political (he wouldn't come out to his parents until much later in life). A few people in KDP offered some solace, including Annie, who came to Michael's memorial service. Nevertheless, Gil wrote, "following [Michael's] death, I felt even more alone than ever before. The majority of KDP comrades didn't know how to respond to my grief since Michael was my gay lover and not my girlfriend or spouse. . . . Had there been a gay Filipino organization . . . , I could at least have gathered some support and understanding for my grief."

Though gone too soon, Michael would have another part in Gil's unfolding story. After the anti-bicentennial parade, Michael had to return the parade banner to a man who was staying at a hotel on Polk Street. Gil went along. Michael introduced him to the man, Juan Lombard, who opened the door to receive the banner. Gil was in love with Michael, so he didn't pay much attention to Juan. Juan didn't live in the city, and Gil didn't think he would see him again.

In November of the same year, Gil, still grieving, decided to go to Monterey for a solo getaway. He had always appreciated the beauty of California's central coast. Decades later, he recounted it clearly: "There were all the windswept cypresses on the cliffside. The ocean breeze, the gentle surf, the white caps. Just gorgeous. Very peaceful just sitting on the rocks and looking at the moss." Looking past the coastline, Gil pledged that he would continue the spirit of social change and revolutionary justice in Michael's memory.

That night, Gil went to the only gay bar in town. People were dancing, but he was content nursing his drink on the back patio with the cabana bar. Gazing at the fire that was burning in the pit to warm the wintry coastal night, Gil was lost in his thoughts. Suddenly, he felt someone standing next to him. His first thought was, "Okay, here we go."

Then the man said, "I know you. You're Gil."

Hearing his name broke his trance.

The man continued, "I remember when you brought the banner from the bicentennial parade. I'm Juan. I know you're thinking about Michael. You're not ready to talk, but here's my number. When you're ready, call me."

Born in 1946, Juan Lombard grew up dirt poor in a Creole community in segregated Louisiana. When he was young, he befriended a kid from a White family who owned a grocery store that the Lombards patronized. The two friends spent a lot of time together until they went to separate schools. "That was when his mom told me we couldn't play together anymore," Juan said. "It was like suddenly you were in a world that you didn't quite understand. It was jarring."

Juan's parents believed that Juan and his siblings could have a better life through education. In an attempt to socialize their children to be academically oriented, Mr. and Mrs. Lombard bought them a set of encyclopedias. For Juan, the pages that included the male anatomy was his "source of eroticism." Masturbating to these images was his first inkling of his sexuality. Juan confessed that he "used it [the encyclopedia] a whole bunch of times that it got yellow."

The encyclopedias did not fail in their academic purpose; Juan earned a scholarship to Xavier University, a Catholic college in New Orleans. Growing up with a vibrant civil rights movement had already predisposed Juan to social justice, and college radicalized him as it did so many young people at the time. Student protests at Xavier exacerbated the tensions between the White nuns who ran the university and the largely Black student population. Juan and his friends started a student newspaper at Xavier to cover the protests, which resulted in the religious order's relinquishing the college presidency to a layperson. Juan is still very proud that the newspaper has continued to this day.

After Xavier, Juan was drafted into the Marine Corps during the Vietnam War. "You couldn't avoid these issues because they personally affected you. There were demonstrations and people were in the streets pretty much most of the time." He didn't end up going to Vietnam; instead, he ended up in Monterey, conveniently close to San Francisco, the hub of gay life on the West Coast.

That was how Juan met Gil again in that bar. Juan said, "When I first saw him, it was lust. I saw his shape and I was like, 'Wow. This is nice.' [laughs] The other part comes later. I admired him for what he was doing because we were both politically involved. There was a certain attraction that goes beyond the physical. I felt I could grow with that person." That night, Juan was biding his time because "[Gil] was going through a tragic situation." But not too long after, Gil called him. And the two started dating.

At first, Gil wanted a closed relationship, but Juan had grown skeptical of monogamy. In our interview, Juan, now approaching seventy, said he "still thinks there's a validity to [open relationships]. It's good to experience other people sexually." War and the failed Nixon presidency plunged the nation into a deeper loss of faith in long-held traditions. The institution of marriage was not immune. After waves of feminism, even many straight people considered marriage more as a patriarchal institution than an inevitable requirement of adulthood.

Reflecting on that time of sexual liberation, Gil understood that he was "modeling after the heterosexual relationship" when he asked for monogamy. It had worked for a little while. Gil relented. "How do you define a gay relationship?" he began asking himself. "Should it be the norms?" Gil eventually came around to Juan's point of view that sexual experimentation and commitment were not incompatible. By the mid-1980s, Juan decided that he had had enough experimentation and was ready to close the relationship. But Gil was just starting.

"I did the switch," Gil said in our interview.

Juan quickly added, "I was like 'What?' But I cared about Gil. If that's what he needed, then I was going to support it."

In 1985, Gil and Juan took a break in their relationship. "A classic seven-year itch," Gil remarked. Gil also wanted a respite from his political work. As conservative forces began to consolidate under the Reagan administration, many leftist organizations, including KDP, were going through an existential turmoil. He moved to Hawai'i. "I went there with the intention of never continuing to be a strong activist, gradually phasing out," he said.

Despite his political connections with some gay men, his sense of responsibility as a KDP leader kept him from fully exploring the gay community in the Bay Area. In Honolulu, Gil made up for lost time. "This is Kalakaua Avenue [the main thoroughfare along Waikiki Beach] in '85. It never looked so good, with all those gay bars," said Gil. "I got hooked into that entire social scene. Really, my gay identity flourished."

It took no time for Gil to become a fixture in the gay community in Honolulu, which he jokingly described as "the imperial court system." He engaged in a series of "affairettes" during his time in Hawai'i, his longest (at four months) being with "the imperial prince," a "Portuguese-Hawaiian cutie." Brent Milburn, the first man he dated on the island, helped Gil find a job at the Life Foundation, an AIDS service organization in Honolulu. At the time, the Life Foundation was run by volunteers to educate and advocate for the community about the virus, which took slightly longer to reach Hawai'i from the Mainland.

"After two years, the organization wanted to open their day-to-day operations," Gil recalled. "I ended up being their administrator, but I was a one-man staff. Oftentimes I ended up being a crisis counselor on the phone. People would walk in off the streets in wrecked conditions. I was jumping from the frying pan into the fire. You really had to learn like this [snaps fingers]." While this was the kind of intense community work he had tried to eschew, his many years of community organizing had equipped him with transferable skills. "I was able to talk with them. 'Are you in touch with a doctor? Are you in a relationship with someone? What's your circumstance?' All the fundamental questions, the basic social service questions. You provide them with knowledge, so they know what to do. Knowledge, attitude, behavior. I didn't know it at that time, but that was the theoretical construct I was working with, which is the same thing when you do political organizing."

While the community work consumed his waking hours, this time at least he could better combine the personal and the political. The "imperial prince" he was dating moonlighted at a bar in the red light district. Gil still remembered the bar vividly: "A genuine dive bar, in this ruddy corner of the red light district. It was like a picture of the 1950s in its heyday. Leopard skin wallpaper, beautiful mahogany bar top with padded leather, with old copper rivets holding them in place. Pin-up pictures of these men on the wall. It was also where all the prostitutes and transvestites came in on break and got loaded, their shoot-up place." Through this connection, Gil provided prevention education to this high-risk population. It was a valuable experience that he would later take to his AIDS work in LA.

He and Juan had separated for about three years, when Gil turned forty. Juan went to Honolulu for Gil's birthday, but he was also intent on having a "come to Jesus" conversation. Gil had had his fun, but Juan wanted a decision: "Either we cut ties, or we get back together." Gil chose Juan, because he realized that no matter which man he was dating in Hawai'i, he was comparing each to Juan.

In 1988, Gil relocated once again, this time to LA, where Juan had settled. The next year, Gil went back to Hawai'i to visit his friends. His vacation coincided with Prince Kūhiō Day, one of two holidays in Hawai'i dedicated to its former royalty. "That was hell of a lot of fun," Gil said. "I got to ride in the parade." Later, as he was partying with his friends, he met one of the biggest drug dealers in the state and "ended up going on a coke binge" (the powder this time, not the soft drink). "I've never done coke before in my life," Gil recalled. "This was, 'Yeah, what the fuck. Go ahead.' He's providing it for free."

One morning, after he returned to LA, Gil "woke up and just felt terrible. I felt like I had the flu. I was cold. I was sweating. I had a fever. I was nauseous. I had a headache." Gil went to the Gay and Lesbian Community Services Center to get tested for HIV.

In those days, people had to wait a week for test results. Gil remembered that people in the waiting room—some waiting for their test, others for their results—were always distant and kept to themselves. The only ripple of emotion came when a person came out of the room with the light step of someone who had tested negative, spared for a little while longer. The mood returned to somber when the counselor called the next number. As the door shut, each person in the waiting room returned to their individual fret.

The person with the number before Gil came out with a light step. "Then," Gil said, "the counselor called my number."

> I walked into his office. He shut the door. He said, "Have a seat." He was on the opposite side of the desk. He asked me, "Well, what do you think the result is?" I paused. It was a point of admission, and not acceptance yet. But I began to admit, "I'm positive." He said, "Yeah."

My life stood still momentarily. Too many things flying around. What do I tell Juan? How do I tell my family? Is he going to leave me? Who do I call? What do I do next? He asked me if I was okay. I said, "Yeah, yeah, yeah." I walked out of counseling. I was oblivious. I was just walking straight to the door. I knew then, when I opened that door, I was stepping into a brand new world.

When I asked Gil how he shared this news with Juan, he couldn't remember. He was so surprised by his lapse of memory—after all, it was his primary preoccupation of this "brand new world"—that he asked me to pause the recording so he could think about it. Then he said that we should ask Juan.

A month later, when I interviewed both of them together, Gil remained befuddled by his memory loss. "I don't know if part of it was the wanting to blank it out because it was so traumatic," he offered. Juan's memory was sketchy, too. But Juan knew one thing for certain: "There was never a thought about dropping the relationship." He still admired Gil, and he wasn't about to leave him for "a mistake." Juan's brother had died of AIDS at twenty-eight. Juan himself worked in the AIDS ward in LA County. "There's a certain part of me that understands this is part of what the community has to go through," he explained. "We all have to be part of it, even though I thought somehow we could escape that. Didn't I pay enough? How much more do I have to give up for it? That's what was disappointing about it."

That neither Gil nor Juan remembered *that* conversation surprised me. After all, this was the most critical moment in their relationship. They could recall lesser events that happened earlier in their lives, or they relished the telling of the more mundane moments of married life. But curiously, that day drew a blank for both. Maybe it was, as Gil said, too traumatic—though there were other stories they told, like those about the deaths of loved ones, that drew tears from these otherwise strong, if weathered, men. Then, what Juan said finally sank in. Among many gay men of their generation, there was an acceptance of AIDS as a constant in their lives. Even if you didn't have the virus, you lived with it in some way. Dwelling on it, not moving on, was equal to paralysis. What is admirable to me was Gil's and Juan's determination not to let the virus take more from them or to change fundamentally who they were: social justice warriors who made a commitment to each other and to the movement.

Their story connected forgotten dots for me. AIDS emerged during a unique period of US history with unprecedented cultural and political transformations, where once-cherished authority and orthodoxy were being challenged on multiple fronts. Asian American studies scholar Glenn Omatsu called this period "a crisis of legitimacy." The years after the 1969 Stonewall Rebellion and the rise of the modern gay and lesbian movement came in the midst of intensifying social movements—feminist, Black Power, anti-war—whose organizing inspired other movements in communities of color, including the Asian American movement. Affirmative action opened access to working-class and first-generation college students, who were exposed to the new ideas fomenting on college campuses. The term *Asian American*—coined during the demand for ethnic studies in California in the late 1960s—and its pan-ethnic concept were about as new as the "gay and lesbian" label. These identities were invigorating to activists who now had the vocabulary to mobilize collective action. In 1973, the American Psychiatric Association removed homosexuality from the list of mental illnesses, and with the ongoing liberalization of state sodomy laws that had begun a decade earlier (Illinois repealed of its sodomy law in 1961, the first state to do so), the pendulum was swinging from suppression to liberation. While many still stayed in the closet, those who could come out did so with a flourish. Same-sex experience was now a basis for an identity—it was who you were, not just what you did. Many rejected conventional relationships and began to experiment with alternatives. In the 1970s, gay clubs in metropolitan areas that had once been hidden and low-key enough that people could sit and talk now became discos, with loud, thumping music. They were both gateways to meeting other gay men and enabling environments for sex, drugs, and alcohol.

"I think the combination affected the sex, too," Juan said. "People would get gonorrhea, and they would just go to the clinic and get penicillin. Then they would go back and do it again. There was no thinking that there might be some consequences down the road. Before AIDS, there was a certain naïvete, like, we could do so many things and be so happy. The sexual pleasure outpaced those other concerns." This sense of invincibility was a euphoric reaction against the repression from the generation before. This was also the age of sex clubs, bath houses, and public sex environments. The gay identity was intimately tied to this freedom to embrace sex of any kind, monogamous or anonymous, without being judged. Gil and Juan's cycles of open and closed relationship did not signal a lack of commitment to one another. Monogamous couples have failed to weather lesser obstacles than the plague they survived. Joyous sex celebrated and validated who they were as gay men. Even as I was coming of age a decade later, it sounded like a utopia.

"A lot of gay people were homeless," Juan continued, "in a sense that they weren't connected to their families anymore." For better or worse, nuclear families had tethered many of them to social conventions. Now unhitched, these gay men felt free to experiment. No one was there to apply the brakes to the experimentation once the crisis hit. Nothing in their history prepared them to think about dire consequences. Nothing prepared them for AIDS.

Tom Callahan, who is married to Dean Goishi, APAIT's founding director, said, "There was this whole thing about being who we wanted to be, being with who we wanted to be, and doing the things that we wanted to do, and things were finally coming together when this ugly disease came on. There was this whole sense of freedom, and then there was this black cloud. It was just a collision. The timing sucked."

It wasn't just men who were sampling tastes of sexual freedom and gender expression. In the mid-1980s, Alice Y. Hom, an LA native, was an undergraduate student at Yale University, where she was beginning to explore her sexuality. She remembered a *Wall Street Journal* article about Yale's "being a gay place." The article, "'Lipsticks' and Lords: Yale's New Look," stirred up quite a controversy and prompted the Yale president to write a rebuttal in the same paper to assuage its alumni.[2] Alice said, "Jodie Foster was at Yale at the time. There was a Yale lesbian group, Yalesbians. There was a group of Yale students who later would write about gay and lesbian subculture, like Sarah Pettit [who went on to found *Out* magazine in 1992]." Alice herself later received a doctorate for her research in the history of organizing among queer women of color. "There was a lot of openness around sexual fluidity, and I felt a part of it. You could go to queer dances and not be perceived as you were gay, because straight people went to the queer dances, too. You would just say you swing. It's this open environment. New wave was very poofy. You had Boy George, you had Prince, you had Adam Ant. You had Annie Lennox dressed in men's suits. It was very gender bending."

In describing his own experience, Ric Parish, cofounder of APAIT, tells a story common to many gay men during that time:

> When I came out, there was no AIDS. I made my debut in 1978 on Castro Street, San Francisco, the tail end of the sexual revolution. I walked down that street, I was eighteen, and I was in paradise. Gay men everywhere, clubs everywhere. Nothing to fear. It was a very different time. There were no sex clubs because you just went to the back rooms in the bars. It wasn't until a year later when I was a student at UC Riverside that we started hearing about this gay cancer that was happening in New York. Everyone was saying, "Oh, it's the S/M [sadomasochism] crowd." I wasn't scared, because I wasn't into S/M. I wasn't doing poppers. I wasn't doing all the things that all the judgments people were making on what it meant to get it [HIV]. And we hadn't seen the full impact. We thought it was just a plot by the Reagan administration, a conspiracy to get us to stop having sex.

According to Ric, it was only when San Francisco shut down all the bathhouses in 1984 that he and his friends knew that "this was for real."

AIDS materialized from a complicated vortex of repression and rebellion and quickly changed the rules. How would you tell those who had cherished such sexual freedom that they must now see bodily fluids as poison, put up barriers in the most intimate of sexual acts, submit to the trepidation and humiliation of testing every six months, disclose their status like a scarlet letter every time they become close to someone? How could any of this not sound like a return trip to the Dark Ages? How could they not be suspicious that this was just another ploy to shame them into normalcy or to blame the victims? After all, those who perpetrated homophobia wielded the same weapon to fan AIDS paranoia.

CHAPTER 2

Universal Precautions

WHEN AIDS BROKE IN 1981, IT WAS INITIALLY CALLED GAY related immune deficiency (GRID), a nomenclature that tied it to all gay men. Nobody knew how it was transmitted, and any casual contact with gay men became suspect. Even when the Centers for Disease Control and Prevention finally settled on acquired immunodeficiency syndrome—AIDS—in September 1982, the phrase *gay cancer* still rolled off many people's tongues. In 1985, former California governor Pat Brown said, "The rise of homosexuality and the acceptance of it has promoted the disease [AIDS] . . . We should make homosexuality like bad breath, not tolerated. It is abnormal. You are talking to a reactionary old man, but that's the way I feel about it."[1] Reactionary punditry like this fanned a forest fire of paranoia that could barely be contained. A 1985 editorial by the *Los Angeles Times* warned against AIDS hysteria and referenced a *Newsweek* poll that found that 28 percent of the respondents avoided places where homosexuals might be present. In a response worthy of *Real Housewives*, women in Beverly Hills counseled each other not to kiss their hairdressers, reported *Newsweek* in 1983.[2] Catholics stopped sharing communion cup at Mass. Morticians refused to embalm people who had died of AIDS.[3]

After scientists determined the transmission routes, early public-health messages emphasized how the virus could *not* be transmitted (e.g., toilet seats, public utensils, handshakes, and door knobs) as much as the actual ways that someone could contract the virus.[4] These implied fears from the public led to the stigma that kept people from doing the kind of things that could contain the epidemic, such as getting tested and seeking medical help.

Such fears were fed partially by the prevalent images of once young, healthy, and beautiful men wasting away in their wheelchairs or deathbeds, their lesioned skin collapsing onto bones like a cloth draping the edge of a table, images that we associated with Holocaust victims or starving masses from faraway lands. Without a cure or effective treatments in sight, infection meant a certain, and often quick, death.

Legislation popped up around the country that stoked these fears rather than actually protecting the population. Some were merely proposed; others passed. In 1986, Proposition 64, which could lead to the quarantining of people with AIDS in California, appeared on the ballot through the efforts by Lyndon LaRouche and his group, the Prevent AIDS Now Initiative Committee, whose acronym unabashedly and unironically spelled PANIC. As late as 1991, LA City councilman Nate Holden proposed legislation to test restaurant workers for HIV. Both efforts failed (Prop 64 by some 71 percent of the voting public).[5] However, in 1987, when a nail salon in West Hollywood canceled an appointment with a client with HIV after a manicurist overheard him telling a friend he had recently been diagnosed with AIDS, an LA County Superior Court judge upheld the business's rights to discriminate against people with AIDS even when the risk of transmission was virtually nil. "There is an extremely small, but nonetheless real, risk of exposure to AIDS from the procedures of a pedicure," The judge pronounced. "An act of discriminatory conduct toward a person afflicted with AIDS is permissible if the conduct is based on a reasonable risk of harm from the afflicted person."[6]

With a touch of hysteria, "extremely small" was amplified to "reasonable risk."

Many in my generation of gay men internalized these fears. When asked how AIDS affected his coming out, Noel Alumit, a writer/actor and AIDS activist, said, "This thing lurking out there, to some degree, affirmed there was maybe something wrong with being LGBT. There was this disease that was coming after us, this impending doom. It colored the way I saw the world and maybe even how the world saw me." Shawn Griffin, an ally to the Asian American AIDS movement in LA, recalled an instance in his youth in Detroit where he recoiled when a friend revealed that he had HIV. His reaction haunts him to this day. In the face of such a grim world, some people turned to addiction (unwittingly putting themselves at higher risk for HIV infection), and others were trapped in sexual paralysis or even driven back to the closet. Irrational fears could be overcome, though. If doom was impending, people like Noel and Shawn decided to meet it head-on, using activism as an antidote to addiction and helplessness.

Perhaps no group revealed the zeitgeist of AIDS panic in those years better than the medical community. These were people of science in healing professions, yet they, too, were susceptible to the irrational fears. Some brave souls stepped up and entered rooms where others hesitated to tread; many became AIDS workers and activists. A handful of people I interviewed started their careers as nurses, social workers, physical therapists, dentists. To do the right thing, they broke ranks. They remembered other nurses who questioned if they had to take care of people with AIDS, dentists who declined patients, and doctors refusing to acknowledge AIDS as a cause of death in death certificates.[7] In LA, both the American Red Cross and the American Heart Association tried to convince their trainers that it was safe to give CPR classes to the public and there was no evidence that the virus could be transmitted through practicing mouth-to-mouth resuscitation on a mannequin.[8] The state of California produced a series of videos to educate mental health providers—a profession that had stopped categorizing homosexuality as a mental illness only a decade before—about how to counsel people with AIDS. Ric Parish, APAIT cofounder, remembered a Korean doctor questioning whether a patient, for whom Ric was making the referral, was actually Korean. In his disbelief, the doctor told Ric that there were no gay Koreans and thus no Korean person with AIDS. "He [the patient] must be Japanese," the doctor concluded.

Yet the AIDS movement couldn't have been possible without those who were in the helping profession. They offered skills about caring for the ill, navigating complicated bureaucracies, and researching the latest treatment advances. As the weekly funeral counts mounted, they provided emotional support to a community that was quickly being decimated.

In 1983, St. Vincent Medical Center, a Catholic hospital at the western edge of downtown LA, received its very first AIDS patient. Nobody knew what to do. Sally Jue was a medical social worker there at the time. She recalled that the admission had made staff "very nervous." She met with the infection control nurse a few times, and together they developed a protocol. This was the time before so-called universal precautions; that set of guidelines informing health care workers on how to avoid a patient's bodily fluids was not introduced until a couple of years later (and then stayed in place until the mid-1990s). The hospital decided to put this patient (we'll call him Carmelo) in an isolation room and post infection-control signs inside and outside the room. "Nobody was allowed to enter his room without wearing a gown and gloves and a mask," Sally recalled.

Sally soon learned Carmelo's story. An immigrant from Argentina, Carmelo was nineteen when he heard a rumor of a gay bar somewhere outside of Buenos Aires. For a month, he drove by the bar repeatedly and staked out the bar in his car, watching people going in and out of the establishment. Finally, he had the courage to step in. Once inside, he was disappointed. Men were talking to and dancing with women; everyone looked heterosexual. Later in the evening, though, the staff locked the doors and drew the blinds. Men and women switched partners to be with their own gender. The place turned into a gay bar. Carmelo became a regular.

Once, a cousin of Carmelo's saw him coming out of the bar and told Carmelo's father. At this news, Carmelo's father disowned him and cast him out of the house. As it was the 1970s, news about gay communities forming in the US prompted him to take a chance and come to LA. He didn't know any English then, and without a support network, he turned tricks on the street to make a living. He would soon meet and engage in longer relationships with "benefactors." These men mentored him and helped him acclimate to his new country. With their help and his increasing command of the English language, Carmelo landed a job with an insurance company and was on his way to independence. That was when he found out he was HIV positive. He was still on probation at work and didn't have any health insurance coverage yet. Undocumented, he had limited options and couldn't afford to stay too long at St. Vincent's. Anyway, the hospital didn't have the capacity to help a patient with pneumocystis pneumonia, one of the earliest and most common manifestations of AIDS. As Carmelo's condition became more stable with some care, the hospital was in a hurry to transfer him to another facility.

During one of Sally's visits with Carmelo, he became visibly upset and started to cry. Sally reached out her hand to comfort him. Her hand was bare; she never thought she needed to wear a glove or take most of the precautions to be in the same room as Carmelo. As her hand was centimeters from his arm, almost feeling his hair on it, Carmelo jerked his arm away. He sobbed even harder.

"I'm sorry," he said. "I didn't mean to offend you. You meant to make me feel better, but I don't know how this disease is transmitted. I don't want you to touch me and possibly get this from the sweat on my arm because you've been so kind to me. If anything happens to you, I just couldn't . . ." His voice trailed off.

At that moment, Sally thought, "Oh my God. Here this man's life is totally falling apart, and he is concerned about me. I need to do whatever I can to help him."

She found out that Harbor/UCLA Medical Center, a county facility, had been admitting people with AIDS. She made arrangements to transfer him. Carmelo needed to be transported by an ambulance because he was breathing with the help of an oxygen tank. His friends chipped in for an ambulance because he couldn't afford it. One of them, Mark, wrote a check for the ambulance company and gave it to Sally, before he headed to Harbor/UCLA to wait and receive Carmelo.

The paramedics came, but when they saw those infection signs outside of Carmelo's room, they turned around and walked out. Sally spent the next hour calling every ambulance company possible. They all refused, despite Sally's pleas. As the transfer was stalling, Carmelo became more anxious. Sally had one last move. She went to the discharge nurse and said, "You need to call in your favors. I know you have a friend at this company that owes you." After learning Carmelo's story, the nurse agreed to help and strong-armed her friend to send a crew. But there was another hiccup. The check that Mark wrote was made out to a different company, but he had already left for Harbor/UCLA. Sally couldn't let the only ambulance that was willing to take Carmelo slip away. "I thought, 'You know what? Fuck it. It's only seventy-five dollars.'" Without telling Carmelo, Sally paid for the ambulance.

With that, Carmelo was on his way. Sally never saw him again, though she received a note from him a month later. He fought on to live another six months. When death was certain, it was the quality of mercy that mattered. The actions of Sally and his friend Mark gave weight to Carmelo's life. In return, his life inspired Mark to go back to school to become a nurse and Sally to volunteer for AIDS Project Los Angeles (APLA), where she supervised other volunteers in bereavement counseling.

In 1984, Sally became APLA's seventh staff person and the first Asian American to be hired. By the time she left the organization ten years later, APLA's staffing had ballooned to more than 130. But in the early days, it was all hands on deck. Hired on initially as a social worker, she was responsible for crisis intervention and support groups. Sally was also giving HIV education presentations and public testimonies. She even started a hospital liaison program and a home visitation program. "I went to a million meetings," she said.

As the only Asian American on staff, Sally took it upon herself to reach out to the local Asian American community. AIDS was not on the community's radar—nor were gay men, for that matter. Official AIDS incidence data at that time lumped Asians in the "Other" category. Sally suspected that even if the incidence rate was low among Asians, AIDS could spread in that community like wild fire if not carefully contained. She was desperate to reach gay Asian men. She had plenty of gay friends, but none was Asian American.

Margaret Endo Shimada was just out of college with a master's degree in social work. With ink barely dried on her diploma, Margaret was hired as the residential treatment director for the Asian American Drug Abuse Program, overseeing an eighteen to twenty-four-month treatment program for drug users. She quickly got a call from Sally.

"I didn't know her," said Margaret. "She said she was with APLA. I've heard of them, but it was a really small organization at the time. She said she wanted to come talk to us about this epidemic that's going to be hitting us very soon, and because it was more pervasive with drug users, she thought we should know about this. I was like twenty-three. I was really naïve and I was like, 'Hmm, are you sure?' Because we haven't heard anything.'"

Sally met with Margaret and her staff. To Margaret's surprise, Sally launched into a safer-sex presentation. "I'll never forget," Margaret said. "She pulled out a banana and put a condom on it. She said, 'I need to teach your residents how to practice safe sex.' She was so passionate. Then not too much happened, to be honest, because that was the very early stage. It was not talked about in the API community much."

Margaret would later learn much more about the epidemic when she became the very first clinical mental health counselor at Asian Pacific AIDS Intervention Team in the 1990s. But in the mid-1980s, she was at a loss as to what to do with the information that Sally was imparting with such urgency. For Sally's part, her presentations in those early days of the epidemic were made to mostly well-intentioned people like Margaret.

One of these presentations finally hit pay dirt. She didn't find a gay Asian man, but she did locate a White psychiatrist at Kaiser Permanente who was dating one. This man and his Asian partner were also members of Asian/Pacific Lesbians and Gays. "You have to come and talk to this group about this," he told her. Sally's presentation fell flat to A/PLG members, but it was still a turning point for her quest, not least because she met Dean Goishi, who, unbeknownst to him at the time, would soon become the patriarch of the Asian American AIDS movement in LA.

CHAPTER 3

A Rumor of Plague

I N THE MID-1980S, DEAN GOISHI HAD JUST QUIT HIS JOB MANAGING the office of an insurance company. In his early forties, Dean was trying to figure out his next move (figure 3.1). He was somewhat active in the gay Asian community in LA through Asian/Pacific Lesbians and Gays (A/PLG), an organization he had cofounded with a group of close friends in 1980. That first generation wanted a space where gay Asian men could build self-esteem for their intersectional identities.

From its inception, A/PLG had a lot of White gay members. The lack of an autonomous community network for gay Asian men was the reason a space like A/PLG was necessary in the first place. These White members were instrumental in swelling the membership rolls in A/PLG's early years. Nevertheless, A/PLG founders had intended to move past this interdependence. In a gay world where their racial identity could be either ostracized or fetishized, they were adamant about reserving leadership positions in A/PLG for its Asian members only. For a while, they experimented with Asian-only "raps" (support groups, in eighties' parlance), even when it was awkward to exclude the White partners.

By 1985, A/PLG had a new group of younger leaders not as invested in the original intentions of founders like Dean. As the first generation of A/PLG leaders handed the baton to the next, the organization was becoming more of a social space, replicating the racial dynamics in the broader gay community. "It was supposed to be always an Asian organization for Asians, and the non-Asians were there as support," Dean said.

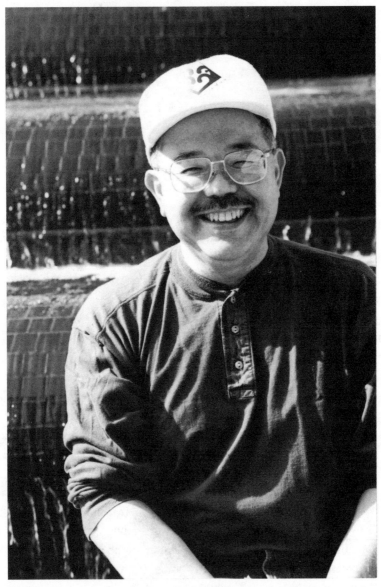

FIGURE 3.1. APAIT cofounder and founding director Dean Goishi, circa early 1990s. Courtesy of Robert Berger.

"But that changed." White gay men became more vocal in the organization, sometimes even being elected as board officers. Older now and a little burned out, Dean and other founding members were starting to fade into the background. Until AIDS.

Sally Jue was invited to give what would be the first presentation about the AIDS epidemic to A/PLG members in 1986. To her surprise, they gave her a reception that was lukewarm, at best. "They were saying, 'Why do we need to worry about this? We're all healthy. Where are the stats on Asians?'" she recalled. When she showed the members the numbers from the "Other" category, under which Asians were collapsed, they dismissed it. They wanted the numbers for each ethnic group or a comparison made between those who were born in the US and those who immigrated to it. Sally left a little deflated. "There was a lot of pushback. They weren't ready yet."

It was not out of epidemiological curiosity that these A/PLG members wanted to disaggregate the data by ethnic groups or immigration status. They were looking for rationalization that the virus only affected *other* groups, even if they fell under the same pan-ethnic umbrella in the organization (Asian/Pacific). It was no different than when the Korean doctor whom Ric encountered dismissed a Korean AIDS patient as Japanese, or when many gay men felt that they were safe because they weren't *those* gay men who injected drugs or partook in kinky sex. Even in the gay community, AIDS was something that happened to *other* people—"the real druggies, the ones who go to Mineshaft in New York [a BDSM gay bar and sex club, made infamous by the photographer Robert Mapplethorpe]," as one of the narrators put it.

There were many reasons for the denial. A/PLG had by then acquired a reputation as a playground for cruising gay Asian men and their (typically White) admirers (crudely called "rice queens"). In this social space, most were not open to such a grim and somber topic. "I don't know if this is racism," Dean added, "but I do think the Caucasian members thought of themselves as saviors or they would take care of the Asian partners and there was not a need to empower the Asian members."

The pushback to Sally's message was also unfortunately reinforced by the scientific community in the early years. AIDS researchers treated this racial group as if they had been given a get out of jail free card during the epidemic. In early 1983, at one of the first AIDS conferences held at the

University of California Medical Center in San Francisco, an epidemiologist told the audience that Asians were likely immune to HIV or at least less likely to contract the virus than other racial groups, based on the fact that there had yet to be any documented cases of Asians with AIDS (the first documented case would not emerge for another three years). The presenter meant to exhort the research community to study this "low-risk" group to learn more about how to contain the virus. In the lay community, though, it gave people a false sense of security. Like a game of telephone, the findings morphed into a rumor circulating at A/PLG and other gay Asian spaces that "there was something in our blood that made us immune," as Dean remembered. Insufficient epidemiological data turned into wishful thinking.

That presentation was widely reported in Asian language media, some of which perpetuated this myth for years, even after evidence clearly contradicted the claim of immunity. From a policy perspective, the narrative that "Asians don't get AIDS" fed into the model-minority myth. The stereotype of orderly and asexual Asians who don't need help gave cover for the ignorance or neglect of policymakers who were doling out already limited resources for AIDS work at the time.

One likely explanation for the low AIDS incidence rate for the Asian population was both ironic and insidious. In a 2003 journal article, "Age and Race Mixing Patterns of Sexual Partnerships among Asian Men Who Have Sex with Men," Kyung-Hee Choi and other researchers found that "HIV prevalence among API MSM [men who have sex with men] may have remained relatively low because higher risk sexual practices occur more frequently within a lower risk API group compared with higher risk non-API groups."[1] In other words, contrary to a popular perception in the gay community at the time that Asians didn't find each other sexually attractive (the corollary of which was White gay men were more natural and desirable sexual partners), this study suggested the opposite, that many Asian MSM kept the virus out of the community by sleeping with each other and not with outsiders who belonged to a higher-risk group.

This was not a conscious self-quarantine. For the most part, decisions around the race of sexual partners were not calculated on AIDS risks. Some community members, like recent immigrants, didn't have a chance to be socialized or introduced into the mainstream gay community yet. The tight-knit nature of these immigrant communities might prevent them from venturing too far from home for this kind of sexual exploration. Having studied the history of gay Asian community formation, I believe there was a more convincing cause for this lack of "race-mixing patterns of sexual partnerships": racism. If Asian men were having a hard time finding sexual encounters with men in other communities, it was likely because, "rice queens" aside, Asian men were not sexually prized in the gay community.

Dean made a similar observation: "The opportunities for gay Asians to engage in high-risk sex were not as great, possibly. We were not sought after by the individuals who could pass the virus to others. That may have kept gay Asians from breaking out. I'd like to think that gave us time to get AIDS education out there to prevent Asians from engaging in high risk behavior."

Oscar de la O, the founding director of Bienestar, an AIDS service organization in the Latino community, recalled a similar line about overweight people. Early on, Oscar heard a clinic staff member say at an education forum that overweight people were not at risk for HIV. Oscar said, " At the time I thought, 'Great, I'm not at risk.' Later, of course, you come to understand that it was the ignorance, the prejudices, that was being disseminated." Could "no fats, no fems, no Asians" truly be a bulwark against an encroaching epidemic? Like I said, ironic, insidious.

The rumor that Asians could be immune to the virus did change *some* people's mind about their desirability. In their article "HIV/AIDS and the Asian and Pacific Islander Community," Deborah A. Lee and Kevin Fong found that after the revelation at the 1983 AIDS conference, "personal ads soliciting Asian men for relationships substantially increased. Some concluded that this happened because white men assumed that they would be safe from the disease if they had Asian partners. Myths, stereotypes, and misinformation, such as the belief that Asian men were immune and lived clean lifestyles—free of drug or alcohol abuse—may have led to social/sexual partnering that possibly helped spread AIDS from mainstream gay community to Asian gays. Asian men, as well, may have endangered themselves by being misled by the popular opinion that they could not be affected by the virus."

Without good data to shed light on their risks, A/PLG members were comfortable in the dark. Some reasoned that if AIDS was such a danger to them, surely some members would've been affected by then, and they would know. There probably were. And they might not know. People who became sick might stop coming to A/PLG. But as Dean found out, you might not know until it was too late.

Dean had a "bar friend" whom he often saw at Mugi's, a rare dive bar where gay Asian men hung out, in what is now the Thai Town part of Hollywood. Dean learned that this friend had contracted HIV. In 1986, that friend was taken to the hospital, and he never left it. "He died there," Dean said. "I found out later that he was also a friend of one of my best friends. And he never disclosed to him that he was ill, either. Nobody knew how serious the illness was." The other friends in Dean's circle all found out about his death independently, and they never discussed his illness with each other. Some in this core group didn't even know the others were friends with him until a postmortem discussion at a get-together. "We didn't know how intertwined his relationship was with each of us," Dean said. This was illustrative of the looseness of the gay Asian network at the time. Spaces existed, like A/PLG or Mugi's, for gay Asian men to find and talk to each other, but these conversations seldom ran too deep.

In my last book, *The Making of a Gay Asian Community*, I talked about how both the stigma of homosexuality and racism in the gay community kept Asian men from becoming intimate—emotionally or sexually—with one another. Dean shared a cultural explanation. "Another part of it was our embarrassment. One, you're not supposed to ask for help. In Japanese, there is a concept of *gaman,* or persevere. You're strong because you don't ask for help. And the other, how do you offer help without embarrassing that person, especially when he hasn't disclosed the fact that he needs help?"

This man's death awakened the group. In 1987, that first generation of A/PLG cofounders established the AIDS Intervention Team (AIT) as a working committee within the organization. In addition to Dean, AIT founding members included Douglas Chin, Herb Dreiwitz, Roy Kawasaki, and Tak Yamamoto. "We decided that we were going to divvy up who we can contact to find out more about HIV and AIDS," Dean recalled. "We would attend workshops that other organizations like APLA [AIDS Project Los Angeles] and Shanti offered." They started exchanging medical information, and they visited and volunteered at hospices to get a better understanding of what people went through at the last stages of the disease. That was another wake-up call. "We realized we needed to deal with death and dying," Dean said. The wave was coming—later than for other communities perhaps, but, as this committee of new AIDS activists came to realize, it would soon engulf them, too.

"It was all self-taught," said Dean, "either by members who were already involved with hospice or medical care or by members who had gone to workshops at other organizations and brought the information back to us so that we could be more effective in how to care for our members who were HIV positive. We had to learn, and we didn't care who was going to teach us." While these workshops from mainstream AIDS service organizations were a good start, they weren't enough to break through the apathy of A/PLG membership. "They were not appropriate for Asians because they just didn't address Asian cultural issues about embarrassment and death and dying," Dean went on. "It was all very Western. They also never mentioned Asians."

Dean turned to two people for help. The first was Sally Jue. From her work experience at APLA, Sally codeveloped some of the workshops for AIT and filled in the cultural competence gaps in other organizations' curricula. Because of her social work background, Sally was also instrumental in coaching AIT's early support group for HIV-positive members.

The other person Dean sought out was his friend Terry Gock, who had been an A/PLG member in its early years. When I sat down with Terry for an interview, he told me that all this misinformation and segregation really set the Asian American community back about five years in AIDS prevention. He drew me two circles. In one were gay Asian men, and in the other was the mainstream gay community. The two barely overlapped. It was a Venn diagram that almost wasn't. He did this to illustrate why prevention messages in the gay community almost never reached gay Asian men. The graphic meant that if gay Asian men were to be informed about AIDS risks, they had to do it themselves.

A psychologist who had been active in the American Psychiatric Association (APA), Terry's first involvement in AIDS work came in 1984, when he helped the state of California plan and review a series of videos to educate mental health providers on how to work with people with HIV and AIDS. "In those days we had VHS [video cassette tapes] training mental health professionals on HIV," Terry said. "There was so much unknown, so much fear that people didn't want to help. They were saying, 'We don't know what to do with these people with AIDS.'" Terry and his colleagues tried to make a case that AIDS was not that different from other terminal illnesses. The resistance, he believed, had just as much to do with people's hang-ups that many who were afflicted were gay. After all, it had been only a decade earlier, in 1973, when the APA made a compromise to remove homosexuality from the Diagnostic and Statistical Manual of Mental Disorder, a diagnostic tool that mental health providers still rely on, and replaced it with "sexual orientation disturbance." Many APA members still retained their biases. The videos that Terry worked on tried to "humanize" these gay men with AIDS (and by extension, lesbians and gay men in general) by explaining some of the challenges they had in confronting a deadly disease.

Terry said, "We were basically saying, you need to understand a little more about gay culture, and how that impacts how [gay men] deal with this disease: the shame, the fear of the unknown, the lack of the general support that other people may have in times of life-threatening illnesses. Some of them are not even out to their parents or their family. They may not have anyone who takes care of them." In other words, AIDS phobia and homophobia are intrinsically entwined, even though we as a society had begun to back away from referring to AIDS as "gay cancer." This became a prevalent approach to raising AIDS awareness; many early workshops on AIDS education incorporated gay and lesbian sensitivity to prime audience to become more receptive to life-saving information.

Terry was well connected in both public and nonprofit sectors, and he was well respected in the broader Asian American community. With both professional and community creds, Terry, along with Sally Jue, was poised to help Dean grow the AIT beyond the confines of A/PLG.

In its first months, AIT directed its energy only toward A/PLG members. They did not promote their PLWA (people living with AIDS) support group outside of their membership or try to find other gay Asian men who were not already part of A/PLG. Dean admitted that "initially, the definition of community was A/PLG members." He remembered helping members who were immigrants in LA by themselves, including a Japanese national who, in his weakened state, had to sleep on the living room floor so that he could open the front door to people he knew were coming to help him without having to walk too far. Other Asian members were not jumping to get involved. Those who had come forward in the support group were White members. "They had partners who were Asians," Dean said. "We were trying to protect the Asian partners from contracting HIV. As far as I know—and I don't know if it's because we were just lucky—the Asian partners were not converting to HIV positive."

Early on, the committee included at most fifteen A/PLG members,. They were spread across six subcommittees, like fundraising and education, with many of them "doubling up as chairs for each of [the subcommittees]." The group held fundraisers not only to raise money for their activities, but also as a way to sneak in AIDS information to unsuspecting members at these events. In addition, core AIT members started working with other AIDS service organizations to provide volunteer and language support.

In the summer of 1987, encouraged by both Sally and Terry, AIT made its first foray into the broader Asian American social service sector so that they could harness the resources and networks of the burgeoning community. They chose to lobby the Asian Pacific Planning Council (APPCON) to institutionalize an HIV/AIDS committee. APPCON was a conglomerate of nonprofit organizations serving the Asian American community in LA. Many APPCON member agencies were relatively small nonprofits that served ethnic-specific populations. APPCON was a place where these agencies could find collaborators in order to ask for larger grants or to have a louder advocacy voice. The establishment of the HIV/AIDS committee would legitimize AIDS as an important cause, on par with other community issues. More than just a symbolic gesture, the committee would also provide a platform for AIDS activists to educate APPCON member agencies and commit them to consider HIV/AIDS in both their advocacy work and collaborative funding.

Terry remembered that there was initial resistance within APPCON because they did not know who Dean and A/PLG were or they had mistaken assumptions about the size of the Asian American gay and lesbian community in LA. Sally recalled this exchange with some APPCON leaders:

You know how people chit chat before a meeting starts? When they asked me how my weekend was, I said, "Oh, well, I had a really interesting weekend. I got invited to the Asian/Pacific Lesbian and Gay fundraiser!" And they said, "We've never heard of them! We don't have any gay organizations in our community." Yeah, you do! "Well, it must have been a really tiny organization." No! No, it has a pretty large membership. In fact, there were about a hundred people at that fundraiser, and they'd be like, "A hundred gay Asians?! No way. They couldn't be all Asians. We've never met any!" I said, "They weren't all Asian/Pacific Islander. Maybe thirty of them were White, but the rest were Asian!' 'Oh, they all must have been American-born." No, actually they told me that maybe 75 percent of their Asian/Pacific Islander membership are immigrants! I mean, it was just really interesting looking at the denial or the lack of exposure. . . . I told Dean later, "The bottom line is, you need more visibility."

Dean had his share of experience with community denial about both HIV/AIDS and gay men. He recalled approaching a nonprofit organization in Chinatown to ask if they could make a presentation to their staff. The executive director told them, "We will listen to your presentation, but there are no gay Chinese. Therefore, you really don't need to come to talk to us about gay issues."

In the 1980s, Terry—just one gay Chinese immigrant whom these providers had known for years—was already active in APPCON, having chaired its mental health committee. He was a known entity, but he was afraid that would not be enough to combat this indifference. So he helped the group gather more allies among the APPCON gatekeepers. One was Royal Morales (Uncle Roy, as he was affectionately called), a founder of Search to Involve Pilipino Americans and at the time the director of Pacific Asian Alcohol and Drug Program, under Special Service for Groups (SSG), a nonprofit that would soon be instrumental in the growth of AIT. When I asked Terry how he got Uncle Roy to back the HIV/AIDS committee proposal, Terry said, "Uncle Roy was Uncle Roy. He was an advocate and a champion. Social justice was in his blood."

The other key ally was Ford Kuramoto, whom Terry had met in the early 1980s when both of them served on the advisory committee for the counseling department of the Gay and Lesbian Community Services Center. Ford would later become the director of the National Asian Pacific American Families against Substance Abuse. At the time, he was working for the LA county Department of Mental Health, running its Hollywood Mental Health Center. In this role, he became intimately familiar with the havoc AIDS was wreaking in LA at one of its epicenters.

Terry said, "We needed the credibility of a bunch of people in order for them to give us a chance to prove this is an issue, that AIT wasn't a wacky group, that they didn't have to be afraid of these people." After a few months of organizing and now with backing from Ford and Uncle Roy, they were finally able to get on the agenda for an APPCON board meeting in late 1987. The day of the presentation, Dean made a grand entrance, wearing hospital gown, face mask, gloves and goggles—the fashion of universal precautions. He was barely recognizable, even to those in the room who knew him. Sally pointed out that "he was making a point of the isolation, the fears, and the misinformation." It was shocking to everyone in the room, except for Sally, who had seen Dean perform in drag to Nancy Sinatra's "These Boots Are Made for Walking" at an A/PLG fundraiser. The get-up was tame in comparison, and it was not entirely unexpected.

Diane Ujiiye, another ally and a staff member at the Asian American Drug Abuse Program, took part in the APPCON presentation. She had been active in the APPCON's drug, alcohol, and tobacco committee. I was struck by those providers in the field of substance abuse coming to the forefront to be allies in the AIDS fight. Certainly, intravenous drug users were a high-risk group. People like Uncle Roy, Ford, and Diane had spent their lives countering the model minority myth and advocating for Asian Americans trying to recover from addiction, people who were obscured by their own community, invisible to the mainstream. This was the same fate that had befallen Asian Americans living with HIV. Diane, however, didn't think that always made it an automatically kindred connection. "At that time, Asian American substance abuse counselors had to address their own homophobia," she said. "I felt like many had this attitude: that's not my job. I'll deal with your drug use, but you have to go to APLA or go somewhere else to take care of your HIV needs. But we could work with you about not getting high. We compartmentalized it because we hadn't been trained on how to address the underlying pain and rejection, and all the mental health issues."

The HIV presentation found some sympathetic ears at the APPCON meeting. Sally recalled that Bill Watanabe, then the executive director of the Little Tokyo Service Center, another heavy hitter within APPCON, spoke in favor of the proposal. In the end, the APPCON board voted to establish an ad hoc task force (not a permanent committee) to look into this issue. Terry agreed to chair it. It would take another two years for APPCON to recognize an HIV/AIDS committee, with representation on its board of directors.

With its AIDS work, AIT began to change the insular nature of A/PLG and gave the organization a public face. In its community guide "Asian Pacific Resources in the Greater LA Area" in October 1988, for HIV/AIDS, APPCON identified Sally Jue individually (as the assistant director of psychosocial services at APLA) as well as AIT, "c/o A/PLG." The guide published a laundry list of AIT's programming, including "AIDS-related topical rap sessions, a PLWA support group, a 'buddy program' in conjunction with APLA, AIDS outreach services (such as Asian language translation for other AIDS-related service organizations), an AIDS education program for the Asian community and gay community, legal services program (such as will and power of attorney preparation for PLWA and their significant others)."

Beyond the minority of A/PLG members who contributed on a voluntary basis, AIT began to attract Asian American lesbians and gay men from a younger generation. In 1989, AIT received a $7,600 grant from the California Community Foundation, its first funding from a foundation, based on a proposal Dean wrote with Tak Yamamoto. The grant allowed AIT to develop its own education materials—written in English, Chinese, Japanese, Khmer, Korean, Tagalog, Thai, and Vietnamese—that resonated culturally with gay Asian men. The translations and illustrations for these materials were all done by AIT volunteers. (Other Asian American nonprofits who benefited from this funding stream included Korean Health Education, Information, and Referrals; the Filipino American Service Group, Inc.; and the United Cambodian Community.)

At the end of that year, A/PLG and other APPCON members formed a partnership called the Asian Pacific AIDS Education Project, with SSG as the fiscal sponsor, to submit a collaborative proposal for prevention and education funding to the LA county Office of AIDS. They argued that an approach focusing on distinct ethnic communities was necessary because, as Dean said, "many gay Asians identified with their ethnic group more so than with being gay." The partnership was a strategic decision. On their own, none of the partners served a population broad enough to make them competitive with other applicants. But together, they became the only choice for the Office of AIDS if the county wanted to address the epidemic in the Asian American community. Having these organizations self-organize through APPCON also spared the county the difficulty of deciding which ethnic communities would get its support and saved them from criticism of favoritism. The partners covered many of the major ethnic groups in LA, including Chinese, Filipino, and Korean, with THE (To Help Everyone) Clinic serving the Japanese, Thai, and Vietnamese populations. A/PLG was the only one that was volunteer-run and had not developed an accounting infrastructure to receive a public contract, but it was the only one with any contact with the gay population, a non-negotiable requirement for the county. This occurred just months after APPCON established the HIV/AIDS Task Force. If the Asian American community had been behind in addressing the epidemic, they were playing catch-up at a fierce speed.

Just because these community-based organizations agreed to be part of the Asian Pacific AIDS Education Project with A/PLG, it didn't mean that their staffs were unequivocally on board with the work. As Dean explained, "Many of them still felt that they had no gays in their communities, and it was not an issue that the general communities would engage in. Sexuality was still a taboo subject. They were hesitant to talk about gay issues, and they knew it." A modicum of discomfort would be counterproductive. How could these straight providers educate others about AIDS if they themselves appeared halting or skeptical? So A/PLG contracted Sally Jue to conduct gay and lesbian sensitivity workshops for the other partners.

The subcontracts for A/PLG and other partners were modest by any measure. They paid for about 25 percent of staff time for each partner. The only full-time staff position was the project director. Insisting that the partnership had to be led by a gay Asian man because the gay community was the most affected, Tak Yamamoto lobbied for Dean to be the project director. Herb Hatanaka, SSG's executive director, agreed. Finally, having spent his unemployment accumulating sweat equity in building an AIDS infrastructure in the Asian American community, Dean became a professional AIDS worker. He had said yes only because he thought this would be a temporary position. "I wasn't looking to work in AIDS," Dean said. "It was never about employment for me. I wasn't an activist. I would never march in the street. At that point, a seed was planted in my psyche that this wasn't going to be long-term." Like many other people at the time, he thought a cure or a vaccine was right around the corner. He had faith that the government would marshal all its public health resources to address the epidemic. In what Dean thought would be intervening years, he would just put his skills managing an insurance company to good use with the AIDS Education Project. "I was probably brainwashed by Tak to think that I was the only person knowledgeable enough to lead the project," he quipped. "Little did I know of the negative factors associated with a 'gay' disease, the politics behind HIV, and all that good stuff."

I describe these early AIDS activists like Dean as "first responders." The death of an A/PLG member—alone, despite his connection to Dean and his friends—compelled them to act collectively to protect the community. "I don't know how we process [his death] other than keeping it in our heads that we're going to do something for the community and try our best to help each other," Dean said. "It was a matter of urgency. That helped organize and sustain us."

Those early years were also a war against gay erasure. To get people to recognize the risk of the epidemic in the Asian American community, they first had to get them to admit that LGBTQ people existed among them. By the early 1990s, Dean had become the face of HIV in the Asian American community. He had appeared in Japanese American newspapers, like the *Rafu Shimpo* (based in LA) and *Hokubei Mainichi* (based in San Francisco). His mother, who lived in Fresno, subscribed to both. Once, Dean brought his partner, Tom, whom he had met in 1991, to visit his mother. Approaching fifty at the time, Dean finally came out to his mother on this visit through his introduction of Tom and their relationship. Dean thought he had shown his hand, both professionally and personally, as a gay man. But a day later, while Dean was taking a shower, his mother, without showing any malice toward Tom, asked Dean's lover "to make sure [he] get married." "Find a good girl and marry and have kids," Dean recalled. "It was in one ear and out the other." Apparently, getting people to acknowledge your existence involved more than just telling people that you existed. Dean later recalled a client who was a Japanese national. When the client's father found out his son had contracted the virus, the father got on the first flight the next day from Tokyo to LA, just to tell his son "that he could not come back to Japan, that he should die here. He couldn't go back because if he did, and people would find out about his status, then they would not be able to marry his sister." It really seemed that in those early days, the closer gayness circled in on the hearths of the Asian American community, the greater the instinct to shoo it away.

Then, a new AIDS activist group formed in New York in 1987 and spread across the US that forever changed the AIDS conversation. It would burst the closet open for LGBTQ people in the early 1990s. Action Coalition to Unleash Power (ACT UP) was the culmination of the resistance that had been fomenting against the neoconservative administration of president Ronald Reagan, who didn't publicly acknowledge AIDS until a press conference in 1985. ACT UP members, mostly White, often gay, carried out civil disobedience against major institutions, from the National Institutes of Health, which allocates funding for medical research, to the Catholic Church and pharmaceutical companies. Theirs weren't just the typical nonviolent demonstrations; ACT UP protests were angry, confrontational, disruptive, graphic, and creative. At times, they were even joyous and fun. They used guerilla theater (like mass die-ins) and fashioned signs and slogans that still resonate with younger generations today. ACT UP focused on how AIDS was an illustration of the inequitable medical system in the US, where not everyone had the same level of access to health care. Practicing a radical democracy, its structure was essentially anarchist; everyone who participated, whether for the first time or the hundredth, had a voice. Made up as a network of committees and caucuses, ACT UP members could nimbly coalesce around issues related to AIDS. ACT UP ushered in a new way of grassroots organizing based on challenging power rather than trying to get a seat at the table. While this style wouldn't spark an interest for Dean and his circle, many younger LGBTQ activists in the Asian American community found it invigorating. Some began to volunteer for AIT in the late 1980s. Before this, AIT already had a tenuous relationship with A/PLG, the organization from which it had sprung. In 1991, something happened that would merge many young activists with the earlier generation of "first responders." This merger eventually forced a break between AIT and its parent.

CHAPTER 4

Fuck That

THE HIV TEST, WHICH DETECTS ANTIBODIES TO THE VIRUS, WAS approved in March 1985. In 1986, the medical group that Ric Parish was working for began administering the tests to patients who wanted it.

"Somebody convinced me to take the test. Bad idea," Ric said, laughing. He was drawn by the novelty of it, and he didn't consider the possible result. "Before I knew it, the nurse came back later that I was positive. It was . . . earth-shattering. I didn't know what to do. I didn't know where to go. I didn't have the infrastructure to handle the result." Neither did his workplace. Focusing mostly on workers' compensation cases, they couldn't offer any support to people like Ric, who had to deal with a grim prognosis. The doctor told him he had two years to live. "And that was being hopeful," he added.

The death sentence didn't leave Ric with a lot of options, and he lived his life "according to that reality." "I shut down," he said. "I hid. I went into a self-destruct bender. I was drinking, and using, and doing all the things you're not supposed to do. Because I believed them. In those days, people with AIDS looked like people in concentration camps: emaciated, Kaposi's Sarcoma, purple lesions all over your body. When people learned their friend was HIV positive or had AIDS, they became untouchable. Nobody would talk to them. I remember when people would put on these space suits to visit people in the hospital. It was devastating."

At the same time, he was beginning to lose friends to the disease. "I had gone through probably two phone books full of friends. In those days we didn't have cell phones to store them. I stopped counting at sixty."

When the two-year mark came around and Ric was still healthy, he struggled to find some normalcy in his life. He switched jobs to become a general manager of a Japanese trading company that had just opened its office in LA. The pay was more than decent. In 1990, he even met Sid, "the love of [his] life." But living with HIV was like living with a time bomb. Even if it didn't go off like you thought it would, it could be detonated at any time. Ironically, things fell apart when Ric was offered a job promotion that would transfer him to Noda, a provincial town in Japan.

He explained: "There is this [Japanese] phenomenon called *karoshi*, which is sudden death [as a result of stress]. One of our executives dropped dead at the airport. That's how stressed out he was. None of the Japanese companies acknowledged that it existed, even though they had a name for it. I was on the verge of a nervous breakdown, and I was depressed. I had to make a decision. I had made enough money where I could take a break. So I quit."

It wasn't Ric's first bout with depression since his diagnosis. Ric's therapist told him to "do something constructive around HIV" to get out of his funk. He volunteered as a buddy for AIDS Project Los Angeles. On the evening of September 30, 1991, he was out with his buddy-client at a restaurant in West Hollywood when suddenly, all hell broke loose in Boys Town, and people were spilling into the street. The crowd was moving east on Santa Monica Boulevard, the main drag in West Hollywood, chanting "Out of the bars. Into the streets!" Ric learned that governor Pete Wilson had just vetoed AB101, which would outlaw employment discrimination against lesbians and gay men. Wilson, a moderate Republican who had been elected just the year before, had promised on his campaign trail that he would sign this legislation if it came to his desk. His veto was a betrayal to the LGBTQ community.

That September evening, I was a UCLA undergraduate having just arrived in Washington, DC, to spend a quarter-term in our nation's capital. I had joined my cohort at a Take Back the Night rally in Dupont Circle. Three hours ahead of the West Coast, we didn't hear about the news of the veto until afterward, when we were waiting for our train in a metro station to go home. A group of us made a detour to the California governor's office on Capitol Hill. Being so far away from California, the sheer size of the protest surprised me. Protesters in DC broke into the building, took the California state flag, and burned it. People were arrested on this side of the country. That was how big a deal the AB101 veto was.

Back in LA, as the uproar reached a fever pitch, Ric and his friend found themselves in the stream of the marchers. Ric said, "I remember passing by the Sports Connection, people started coming out of the gym and joining. It was an amazing sight. I didn't know where we were going. I didn't know what we were going to accomplish, but we were letting our voices be known."

The protests would continue nightly for two weeks. The organizing was relatively decentralized. ACT UP and Queer Nation members were involved, but many of the leaders were actually away in DC for a conference (which explained the fervor of the protest I witnessed). Many protesters took to the streets on their own when they found out where people were congregating. After the first night in West Hollywood, demonstrators flooded other parts of LA. Ric went to many of these protests. He was there when they marched through Century City, a few miles west of West Hollywood, headquarters of big law firms and entertainment conglomerates, as well as an open-air mall that catered to the upper crust.

"That was scary," he recalled, "because the police chased us with horses into the mall. They chased some ACT UP members into Neiman Marcus; 'Needless Markup' was what we used to call it. They also knocked down some of the wrong people, some very wealthy shoppers."

He was there at the ACT UP demonstration at the Los Angeles International Airport. Marching through the terminals, the crowd was chanting, "Hey, hey! We're gay! Welcome to LA!" "When you come into LAX, you can see those airplanes out there," Ric explained. "These Southwest [Airlines] flight attendants—the little gay boys—were waving and cheering from the door of the airplane. It was amazing."

Even the activists themselves were surprised by the energy and longevity of these demonstrations. In her book *The Life and Death of ACT UP/LA*, Benita Roth interviewed Walt "Cat" Walker, one of the ACT UP/LA leaders who were in Washington, DC, the night of the veto.

Here we were in Washington DC and we kind of considered ourselves the cream of LA gay activists at this point [laughs]. . . . When we first heard about the veto, we actually said things like 'oh, they'll probably have a big demonstration in San Francisco, but LA won't do anything, especially with us here.' And then we heard that there were these great big demonstrations in LA and it blew our minds . . . especially because the people who were leading and organizing these demonstrations were people who had not been involved in ACT UP. They were a new group of people.[1]

These protests were a promise of great things to come in LGBTQ activism in LA.

That thought occurred to Ric on the first night, when he turned around in the impromptu march and saw a few thousand people behind him on Santa Monica Boulevard. "This is much bigger than any of us here realize," he thought to himself. "This is the spark that will unite activism in Los Angeles."

At one of the marches, Ric saw a group of Asian Americans. One particular "big, stocky Filipino guy" held his attention because he was carrying a sign that read, "Throw Pete Wilson into Mount Pinatubo," a reference to the volcano in the Philippines that had erupted earlier that year, spewing magma for months. As both Filipino and African American, Ric was immediately drawn to this young man and the anticolonial tinge in his message. "I had to go meet him," he said. "Little did I know that this man would eventually become one of my closest friends and allies, Joël Barraquiel Tan."

It was a meeting that changed the course of Asian American AIDS activism in LA.

Joël was an "AIDS geek," but one with a fiery brand. It was no coincidence that the first image Ric associated with him was an angry volcano. When Joël was a high school senior, he argued in his debate class against Proposition 64, the 1986 ballot initiative that would allow the state to quarantine people with AIDS. Joël's sentiments against the proposition were so strong that he remembered this debate as a "seminal moment" in his political development. "I felt connected to the movement," he said.

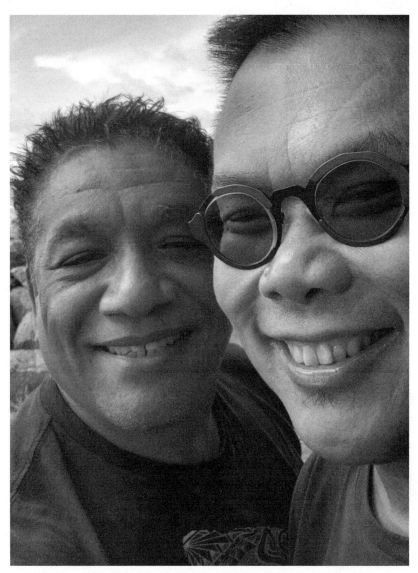

FIGURE 4.1. APAIT cofounders Ric Parish (left) and Joël Barraquiel Tan, in Hawaiokinai, where they both currently reside (2020). Courtesy of Ric Parish.

After high school, Joël eschewed higher education, thinking that everything he needed to learn he could learn from working in the community. He first worked at a transition home for gay and lesbian youth called Citrus House, operated since the early 1970s by the Gay and Lesbian Community Services Center in a house on Citrus Street that had been donated by the city of LA. Joël wasn't even old enough to drink legally, but he was the house manager, working with youth that had been discarded by society. Many of these youth were sex workers. There, he came face to face with the epidemic.

"There was a young man who was diagnosed," he recalled. "He was distraught until one day he came to me and said, 'I'm going to be cured. I'm getting a sex change and I won't have HIV anymore.' That moment has always stayed with me. My entire life, it reminds me of how important the work is. The look of genuine hope on this young person's face when he thought that was possible. It tore me apart."

Another job Joël held before meeting Ric was as a home health-care worker through a nursing service. He was assigned to take care of a man with HIV who had been Mr. Gay Universe not too long before. Joël would take his charge to his appointments at the County-USC Medical Center. "I was carrying this man on my back practically who had been Mr. Gay Universe, into the AIDS ward where he would do his lung treatments for PCP [pneumocystis pneumonia]," Joël said. "He would be sitting there, in a waiting room full of other AIDS patients with IV poles."

He remembered making a pilgrimage to the Castro district, just after high school and with a fake ID, "ready to get my San Francisco gay man's moment on." Instead, he said, the Castro "was nearly deserted, and the first person I ran into at this donut shop was a dude with an IV pole who was just fucking staring at me pissed off. It was so confusing." Born in 1968, just before the Stonewall Rebellion, Joël had grown up thinking gay life would be like "having Sylvester singing 'Mighty Real' always in the background with shirts off and joyful fucking everywhere." "I didn't get that," he said. "I got fucking IV poles. It was the trope of the IVs and the once beautiful men decimated to skeletons. It was a fucking plague war. I wasn't even twenty-one. This was my sexual coming of age. What the fuck?"

AIDS was a "total betrayal" to many young people like him. Joël said, "There's a part of me that feels like HIV cheated me out of a really lush sex life. I feel like I would've been in considerably more gangbangs and all kinds of wild shit if I hadn't been so fucking scared to die." For years, while watching friends and lovers die from AIDS complications, the randomness of infection just made the epidemic so chilling that even when he had "avoided anal sex like a plague," he questioned whether he had "an undetectable strain" of the virus. For someone who had "constantly promoted radical sex positivity" during the AIDS epidemic, the irony that he "was petrified by [his] sexuality" was not lost on him.

As Ric expected, Joël shared a progressive vision that was rooted in their shared Filipino heritage. Joël owed his early politicized consciousness to his mother, who was involved in the anti-Marcos movement in the Philippines. He said, "It's what triggered us having to come to the US in the first place, so I had a clear idea from a young age what colonialism is, what White supremacy is, how Americans have dominated. I wasn't empowered by the gay API movement. In retrospect, they were very much grounded in twentieth century values, and I was already inching toward the twenty-first century. Like they were still, 'I'm gay and Asian.' I'm like, 'I'm queer.'" Ric's mother would tell him stories about the Japanese occupation of the Philippines, like having to bury American pilots who fell dead in their backyard from a B-29 bomber that had exploded in the air. She and her sister were forced to work in a factory and make parachutes for the Japanese colonizers. "So they figured out how to tie the parachutes in a way so that they didn't open," Ric said. "That was her contribution to the war effort [laughs]. They almost got caught. My stepmother was from Sasebo [a fishing village on the island of Kyushu]. She survived Nagasaki because when the bomb went off, they were on the other side of one of the hills, which shielded them from the blast. My brother was in Vietnam. He was a marine. This is the backdrop of where I came from. I couldn't help but have a global vision growing up."

When Ric and Joël met in 1991, Joël had just started a job working at Search to Involve Pilipino Americans, a partner in the Asian Pacific AIDS Education Project, the collaborative that Dean Goishi was directing. Joël became one of those younger people crashing A/PLG who were more interested in its AIDS voluntarism and shunned its social functions. The AB101 protests gave Joël another avenue for his activism. "I threw myself into movement work," he said. "A lot of us who came up that way found our identity and sexuality through movement work as well." Joël soon began to gather others whose sexual identity was also quickened by the unfolding protests.

"I quickly realized that the LGBT movement was clearly about Whiteness," Joël recalled. "It was unconscious of and suffering from its own sense of White supremacy. Looking at the architects of these protests, I just thought, 'Fuck that. I'm going to get my lovers and friends together and we're going to create our own coalition of color.' I stitched together my connections working at the Gay and Lesbian Center and also my own personal networks, like dudes I was dating and fucking who belonged to Gay and Lesbian Latinos Unidos and Black Men's Exchange." That led to the birth of Colors United Action Coalition.

In the aftermath of the AB101 veto, Colors United formed an alliance with ACT UP/LA, Queer Nation, and League America, which Joël described as "the Richie Rich, gay conservatives from the Westside. They brought their Beamers and Benzes to the meetings." Ric remembered those meetings as being tense and rocky. In some ways, these gay Republicans felt most betrayed by Wilson's veto, their sense of entitlement shattered by the denial from a pen's stroke. But even this shared sense of betrayal couldn't sustain the alliance.

The radical politics of White gay men and lesbians in ACT UP and Queer Nation resonated with both Ric's and Joël's families' history of resistance. ACT UP/LA's commitment to research and development (R&D) and cultural productions, as well as Queer Nation's "radical broad sexuality," as Joël Tan characterized it, deeply influenced the political expression of this generation of queer activists of color. Some of the most radical White queer activists from ACT UP/LA, such as Mary Lucey, Gunther Freehill, and Ferd Eggan, would become mentors, allies, and role models for Ric, Joël, and the young HIV/AIDS activists they would soon gather.

Eric Reyes, who met Ric and Joël through Colors United, saw its governance structure—every member being empowered in decision-making, building consensus even if the process was cumbersome and time consuming—as a reflection of the "experiment in radical democracy by White gay radicals in ACT UP/LA and Queer Nation." Even then, activists of color might disagree with some of their direct actions. For instance, when ACT UP/LA was planning an action against Cardinal Roger Mahoney and the Catholic Church, Ric remembered Joël saying, "If you guys go to Mass and stick a condom in my grandmother's face, I'm going to kick your ass." Ric added, "That was at the heart and soul of how we did things differently." Eric explained it this way: "We saw those expression of White gay male rage, at the loss of privilege. These were groups that could do that because they were White. That's not to detract at all from the work that both of those groups [ACT UP and Queer Nation] did, because they did substantially change the American psyche about HIV and the LGBTQ communities." As Colors United began to solidify, they also understood they had to organize separately to lift up the voices of people of color.

Joël organized a contingent of Colors United members—about a hundred, in his memory—to disrupt Creating Change, the annual conference of the National Gay and Lesbian Task Force that was held in LA in 1992. "They were talking about AB101, but there was no discussion about how race was factored in. We walked into the ballroom, all people of color. We were like, 'Nope. You're not having that discussion.'" Urvashi Vaid, the executive director of the Task Force and a South Asian lesbian, tried to placate the protesters. "It was Urvashi," Joël said. "All the White gays knew and loved her. She said, 'I'm an Asian lesbian, too.' And I said, 'No, you're a professional lesbian. You're not in our registry, Boo.' I was so cheeky. Now at fifty, I'm like, 'I was such a punk ass.' But that was the younger generation at the time." Disrupting the mainstream and injecting racial politics—even when the mainstream organization was led by a forward-thinking progressive woman of color—was perhaps necessary in building institutions in LGBTQ communities of color that had been marginalized and neglected. A self-proclaimed enfant terrible, Joël said, "I felt like my job for a while was kicking down doors. In the early part of the movement, my triggering response was 'Fuck that.' That was how we were going to make changes."

Colors United soon grew large enough that it started having race-based caucuses. The Asian and Pacific Islander Caucus decided to organize around HIV/AIDS. Unlike Dean's generation of "first responders," these young activists, influenced by the increasing radicalization of LGBTQ politics, didn't see HIV/AIDS as a single issue but the nexus around which they could develop deeper analysis about broader systemic inequalities, like health-care access and housing and employment discrimination.

Ric explained, "There was this narrative back in the day that gay White men were the first to get AIDS and they were the first to start dying. We challenged that narrative. They were the first to have primary health care, so they were the first to get in and get counted. People of color, women, the transgender community, they were dying on the streets. It took a while for the epidemic to reveal itself. We were in the middle of exploring that, searching in the wilderness of this reality called HIV/AIDS." This collective political education revealed a health-care crisis in America to the young activists. "Everybody has a right to live," Ric continued. "Everybody has a right to be healthy. Why shouldn't everyone have insurance and access to adequate health care, just to stay alive? It's a basic human right. . . . These were not new ideas, but the epidemic shined a light on that and showed us that we really needed to focus on health care as a right rather than a privilege." This fringe idea of universal health care would become the prime battleground of ideological struggles in American politics in the next three decades and counting.

Ric continued, citing Black trans activist Ashlee Marie Preston's idea of "disproportionate realities":

> If you have access, there are certain things you just take for granted, right? And if you don't have housing, you're going to think, "Okay, HIV may not be my number one priority. Getting a roof over my head might be the priority." In order to address HIV in a broader context, there has to be a multiplicity of approaches because not one approach is going to fit everybody. You can't even talk about adherence to HIV medication if you've got a needle in your arm and you can't stop. You can't talk about having refrigerated medication if you don't have a refrigerator, if you don't even have a place to stay.

Similarly, Joël, while at SIPA, collaborated with the Asian Pacific American Legal Center to help undocumented Filipino immigrants with HIV to address their immigration problems. Poverty, housing instability, and immigration status were intrinsically tied to HIV/AIDS. Yet these basic issues didn't figure into the reality of many middle-class or White gay activists or mainstream AIDS service organizations.

Because Joël was already connected with the AIDS Intervention Team (AIT) at A/PLG, Colors United organized to bring their fiery brand of politics to the organization. AIT's relationship with A/PLG was already tenuous. Now, AIT was swelling its membership with people who neither paid dues nor subscribed to its social mission. The influx of these younger activists pushed AIT further in a direction in which it was already crawling: toward separation.

CHAPTER 5

Exit Strategies

I N 1990, DEAN GOISHI WAS FINISHING UP HIS FIRST TERM AS THE director of the Asian Pacific AIDS Education Project. His priority as director had been administrative and fiscal rigor. "You had to develop a good structure, good record keeping," Dean said. "Fiscally you had to be sound. Otherwise funders wouldn't like you." That this was the first Asian American AIDS project in the county also weighed on his mind. "I didn't want to fail and show my disgraceful face to the community," he added. Though shame driven, Dean's focus was laser sharp and unwavering. This attention to infrastructure, in the service of "contract compliance," would explain his institution-building approach later in the movement. For this inaugural project, it served Dean well. The three-year grant was up for renewal that year, and its chances were looking good.

In spite of this, Dean was feeling a bit restless. During the third year of the project, its fiscal sponsor had switched from Special Service for Groups (SSG) to the Asian Pacific Health Care Venture (APHCV). An outgrowth of the health committee within the Asian Pacific Planning Council (APPCON), APHCV was set up to help family clinics in the ethnic Asian communities to become primary-care providers to their immigrant, often linguistically isolated, populations. Established in 1986, it incorporated as a nonprofit organization a year later. It took a few more years for it to gain some experience handling county contracts. Once it did, however, APPCON leaders felt that it was a better and "more pragmatic" fit as a fiscal sponsor for the AIDS Education Project. APHCV was already in partnership with many clinical providers that were already part of the AIDS Education Project, including THE Clinic, Chinatown Service Center, and Koryo Health Foundation.

These advantages didn't pan out as expected. Getting these partners to talk about HIV/AIDS with their clients turned out to be Dean's "steepest learning curve." He ran into the same old wall of homophobia or gay erasure in these ethnic communities. Men in these communities who engaged in unsafe sex with other men were too afraid to seek information about HIV. They might seek care at these clinics without revealing their sexual practices, and providers had to be sensitive to give health information to them without shaming or scaring them away. How could they do that when, as Dean explained, "many of [the providers] still felt they had no gays in their communities"? Even when sympathetic, they were hesitant to bring up the taboo subject.

These sentiments persisted well into the 1990s. Heng Foong ran a program that dispatched interpreters to help monolingual patients with AIDS during a doctor's visit so they could receive accurate life-saving information. She received some feedback from an interpreter who came back from an assignment at Pacific Alliance Medical Center in Chinatown. The interpreter observed that "the physician was so dismissive of the disease. He didn't even want to talk about it." Heng was convinced that was why the patient died so quickly.

Providers in family clinics were already trained to teach the community about other sexually transmitted diseases. The discomfort in discussing AIDS had to do with its association with homosexuality. It wasn't just sex that was taboo; it was gay sex in particular. Lisa Hasegawa, who joined APHCV as an intern before being hired on as an administrative assistant in 1991, added, "It was a time where everybody was just learning the language about how not to be homophobic unintentionally. Those early trainings were about basic awareness, like 'Don't say, "That's so gay."' Those were some really basic stuff. So definitely it was hard to talk about HIV and AIDS, and also queerness."

The homophobia didn't come only from one's cultural traditions. Lisa remembered conversations about whether these ethnic-specific partners had the capacity to carry out AIDS education when "many of those staff were very religious." She remembered a program director at a partner organization who was a minister's wife. To this person, doing family planning in immigrant communities was already "pushing the envelope." "She was a Methodist, and she had said Methodists were the devil to the Baptists," Lisa added, just to underscore how even more severe other Christian denominations could be.

Lisa also wondered if immigrants who were at high risk for HIV would go for help to a provider in their ethnic enclave. Sally Jue had spent most of her early AIDS career looking for this high-risk population. She explained it this way: "The stigma piece was huge. Immigrants preferred going to service providers that spoke their language, understood their culture and were more like them. Well, when it came to Asian gay folks, they preferred to go to White doctors and mainstream HIV service organizations, *if* they could find somebody that they felt understood them culturally, because things would more likely to stay confidential there. And they would feel less judgment than from people from their own communities, because of gay stigma, which was also HIV stigma." The tighter knit the community, the bigger the fear of exposure to people they had to interact with every day. Yet for immigrants who had limited English proficiency, they couldn't go to mainstream providers who didn't speak their language. So they ended up going nowhere at all. "It was a huge gap," Lisa concluded.

As director, Dean felt this program theory of training providers, who were otherwise cultural and linguistic competent, to deliver AIDS education to their respective community was riddled with limitations. Most of the partners were passing out brochures passively or holding workshops at their offices, which Dean described was a "shotgun" approach. Dean wasn't sure if their general outreach was getting to the people in that huge gap that Lisa was talking about. The partners didn't target specific groups within the community, have one-on-one conversations with people to assess whether they were engaging in high-risk behavior, or go to public spaces where these people were likely to congregate. Dean said, "At some point, the county wanted to know how many gay folks were being impacted by our programs, and they would not be able to tell them." Based on the anecdotal evidence Dean was seeing, he felt that immigrant men with limited English proficiency who have sex with men (MSM) "were not getting information and education [about HIV]. They were not protecting themselves." This group—immigrant MSM unassimilated into the mainstream gay community—is what I call the holy grail of AIDS outreach.

The other challenge was that the contract amount wasn't that large. Split among multiple agencies, the subcontract amount translated to about ten hours a week on the AIDS Education Project for each partner. Many of these staff members were assigned other projects, competing for their attention. It didn't even have to be blatant homophobia. If the staff was not that invested in HIV/AIDS work already, that work often fell by the wayside. Dean had to push to get many of the partners to meet the monthly numerical targets set in the contract.

He cited one exception: Search to Involve Pilipino Americans (SIPA). SIPA was more open to HIV work for a few reasons, he believed. First, as ethnic-specific data became available and confirmed what people in the community already knew, the epidemic hit the Filipino community the hardest among all the ethnic groups (the Thai community had a higher incidence rate, but it was much smaller in size). Second, there were many champions in the Filipino American community for the cause, including straight allies. When SIPA set up its AIDS Task Force as part of the AIDS Education Project subcontract, it included Royal Morales, the same Uncle Roy who helped get APPCON to recognize a committee on HIV/AIDS, and other community leaders, such as Meg Thornton (former SIPA executive director), Cheryl Mendoza (who had been a part of the leadership at the Gay and Lesbian Community Services Center and a program officer at the California Community Foundation), Marissa Castro, and Florante Ibañez. They also recruited Gil Mangaoang, who by then had moved to LA and was very public about his status.

This initial AIDS funding helped these community organizations evolve, even if not very perceptibly in the beginning. Eric Reyes succeeded Dean as the next director of the AIDS Education Project. Even though he inherited the same challenges, he maintained that "it forced these very heterosexually oriented organizations to open up and realize that there are people in their community they needed to deal with. Some actually recruited and brought them in [as staff]. That's one of these institutional, secondary effects people don't really think about."

The scope for A/PLG was different. A/PLG contracted Sally Jue to develop a curriculum to train Asian American providers on sexual orientation and HIV/AIDS. In addition to being the full-time director managing the project, Dean often wore his volunteer hat at A/PLG to co-train with Sally. Wearing two hats was not sustainable. Having a new supervisor at APHCV didn't help. Dean held on for a while, but eventually, he decided he was much more effective under the hands-off style of his former fiscal sponsor, SSG. "I was already comfortable with my own abilities, and I really did not need to be managed by somebody who I didn't know that well," he said. Yet he had to put a few things in place before he could walk away.

The reality was that the nature of AIDS funding was changing. As the epidemic matured, funding for prevention was no longer just about community education. More than increasing general awareness and knowledge about HIV/AIDS, funders wanted to see more targeted outreach to high-risk populations to change their behavior. The type of passive outreach that the partners in the AIDS Education Project were doing, Dean foresaw, wouldn't be sustained forever. If they weren't reaching MSM in their ethnic community, how would they demonstrate any behavior change? In 1990, the state released a new funding stream and invited applications that focused on "behavioral modification." This time, A/PLG went it alone. Almost.

With the California Community Foundation grant and the county subcontract under their belt, AIDS Intervention Team (AIT) leaders felt confident that they could now compete for state funding, but none of its members knew how to prepare a state proposal. The higher the funding level, the more complex and technical the application instructions. State proposals often entail hundreds of pages, and experienced grant writers know that it is more about the careful organization of information than the eloquence of prose. On top of that, A/PLG didn't want to involve their old standbys this time.

"We tried to keep Sally Jue and Terry Gock out," Dean said, "because they were going to be reviewers for the state. We didn't want them to be in conflict of interest. They knew the Asian community and all its nuances. None of the other review people knew of our idiosyncrasies."

Strategically, A/PLG benched their most knowledgeable allies to up their inside game. They had to look for help elsewhere.

Naomi Kageyama was in her twenties when she was brought on by SSG to work on development. She had a knack for writing proposals, even though her undergraduate degree was in biology. "I was trying to be the good Asian," she said, referring to her science background. "I realized that was not really my passion." A volunteer stint at the Little Tokyo Service Center had raised her consciousness and changed her career path. At SSG, writing the proposal for A/PLG was among her first assignments. Knowing that data showed that the AIDS incidence rate for Asians was low compared to other communities, Naomi knew she had to be creative, even within the rigid perimeters of state guidelines, if she were to make reviewers understand their needs. "I always thought, if I'm a reviewer, what would get to me?" She said. "You had to rely on stories. I always find ways to add that touch." Along with Paul Chika-hisa at SSG, Naomi worked closely with Dean and began to learn about stories of prejudice and discrimination that the LGBTQ Asian Ameri-can community suffered on a regular basis. They folded neatly into her evolving consciousness of community service.

In 1991, A/PLG received news that their state proposal had succeeded. The agency finally had money to hire their own paid staff to do street outreach and to go to places where MSM might hang out, instead of doing AIDS education to the general public and waiting for MSM to show up at some agency's door. Dean, who was still planning his transition out of the Asian Pacific AIDS Education Project, wasn't avail-able. Besides, approaching fifty now, he knew that he wasn't the ideal candidate to talk to young people at the bars or anywhere where Asian MSM congregated. Fortuitously, AIT had been attracting a steady stream of younger activists. With state funding, A/PLG finally was able to hire their first two outreach staff from this pool: Joël Tan and Ric Parish.

By then, APHCV had moved its office into an abandoned bank build-ing at the intersection of Cesar Chavez Boulevard and Broadway, at the outskirts of Chinatown, affectionately known in the community as the Chinatown Annex. Though by no means a large facility, the building was also the site of several small Asian American community-based organ-izations. The Gay Asian Pacific Support Network held an office for stor-age and hosted their rap (support) group on the bottom floor of the building every month. In 1992, the APHCV staff who worked at the Annex were Dean, Lisa, and Kazue Shibata, APHCV's executive direc-tor. When they were not doing street and bar outreach, Joël and Ric also held their office in the Annex. Lisa and Joël became fast friends, partly because they were close in age. "We were baby activists," said Joël, who still calls Lisa one of his dearest "sisterfriends." Their bond went beyond age, though. Not long after Joël joined the A/PLG staff, Lisa successfully garnered a teenage pregnancy prevention grant from the state for APHCV to provide sex education to young people in the Asian American community. She was promoted from administrative assistant to managing this new program.

Lisa would go on to become a national leader in community development in the Asian American community. In the early 1990s, barely out of college, she had landed an entry-level job at a new nonprofit based solely on the fact that she could take notes and make flyers on a personal computer, a not inconsequential skill at a time when the first Mac Power-Books were hitting the market. Within a year, she was put in charge of managing a state grant. "Little did I know that it was the very first API reproductive health education program in the whole country," Lisa recalled:

> There was no data on high-risk behaviors of Asian young people in
> Los Angeles. That was weird to me. Kazue was like, "Well, duh. Just
> tell your own story." And I did. I was one of those high-risk youth,
> growing up in Orange, hanging out with all the Vietnamese gangster
> boys. When I dated a Vietnamese guy in high school, the Vietnamese
> club scene was crazy. Everybody was having sex with everybody. And
> seven years later, I was working at the Health Care Venture, and
> people were saying that Asian kids don't have sex. I'm like, "What
> planet are you from?" There was a lot of personal storytelling about
> our own sexuality, about our own understanding of what reproductive
> justice meant, and just pushing back on people's discomfort with
> talking about sex. I was the sex lady. We were the ones that were
> boldly talking about sex in the Asian American community when no
> one wanted to talk about it. That's where I found kinship with Joël.

The parallels between reproductive justice and AIDS activism sharpened their political consciousness. Drawing from her own experience as a teenager, Lisa knew her sex education could be reaching young people who might be struggling with their queerness. She said, "In high school, there were quite a few gay and lesbian folks in my fairly close circle. We were all into the New Wave, like the Cure, Duran Duran, and Depeche Mode. I guess there was a part of me that already felt aligned with a more edgy crew. It wasn't that much of a transition to be a part of that world."

Their office discussion led to collaboration. With Joël's help, Lisa included HIV/AIDS in her sex education curriculum. This strategy was controversial. The pushback came not from the community's resistance to discuss sex and its consequences, but from the state and its leadership, the same Republican governor Pete Wilson who vetoed the AB101 bill. Wilson wanted the sex education curriculum to be "abstinence based." Lisa said, "I became active in the fight along with Planned Parenthood and others about the fact that the curriculum was too conservative and we should really be providing much more information about HIV and AIDS and about contraception while we were doing teen pregnancy prevention." After all, sexually transmitted diseases were an essential part of sex education curriculum, and it would be unconscionable to leave out the deadliest STD of the generation. Understanding one's sexuality was key to decisions one would make about how, when, and whom to have sex with. "Abstinence based" was different from "abstinence only," a more rigid federal standard where more topics would be off the table. That small difference gave Lisa and other advocates just enough room to sneak in the information they thought was important for teens to know, while giving lip service to the supremacy of abstinence.

Lisa and Joël were working with overlapping circles of Asian American community organizations, especially the youth-serving agencies through the Service Network for Asian Pacific Youth, another APPCON committee. Some of these organizations were able to streamline their different priorities into joint efforts. For instance, when anti-tobacco public funding started to flood the nonprofit sector, many of these organizations were funded to do substance abuse prevention. To give young people a more well-rounded youth-development experience, these providers cross-trained each other on substance use, sexually transmitted diseases (including HIV/AIDS), and teenage pregnancy. Being tied to different issues forced providers in other areas of expertise to acknowledge HIV/AIDS as an issue that deserved equal focus. For instance, prior to doing AIDS work, JJ Joo was the artistic director of the Asian American Community Teen Theater. He worked with the youth to develop and perform stories linking multiple issues affecting youth, including HIV/AIDS. This was another approach to mainstream the disease.

Building alliance, pushing the envelope, making connections even when funding was siloed—these were just some of the skills that Lisa took with her as she ascended the leadership ladder in Asian American community advocacy nationally. Reflecting on those years, Lisa said, "I certainly connect my introduction to advocacy to HIV/AIDS organizing. And I definitely learned from the best, the best because they were in the hardest situations. It was just challenging for Dean to go into some meeting and face service providers who were just not respectful. And for Joël to be Filipino in a mostly East Asian world. You just learn fearlessness, and that for me was a gift, to always challenge the status quo."

While Joël was finding some camaraderie with APHCV and its network, an internal fissure was growing in A/PLG. AIT volunteers, mostly from Colors United, were increasingly younger and more activist minded. They had a different agenda in joining the group and could care less about the social mission of the parent organization. On the other hand, A/PLG leadership wanted these new volunteers to pay membership dues. Because some in the committee were HIV positive, the AIT group didn't even want to share their membership list with A/PLG, let alone collect dues.

Never mind that the AIT's budget had already eclipsed that of A/PLG and that its AIDS work had finally given A/PLG some visibility in the Asian American community. The leadership was no more committed to fighting the epidemic than when Dean and his circle started the modest offshoot four years ago. Dean suggested that it was a product of internalized racism: "The membership thought their White, or non-Asian, partners could protect them, and therefore, they were safe." This kind of mentality riled the younger generation, as they began to see the impact of the epidemic up close. Joël said, "All these old snow queens. We were so dismissive of them and their fucking Lacoste. . . . It was us young people who was going out to the bars. We were the ones going to the sex clubs. Really it was about recruiting that next wave of activists." They had been impatient about the problematic racial dynamics of the organization or its self-interested insularity, but at least they could avoid A/PLG's social functions. But when A/PLG leaders' indifference started to impede AIT's growth, the AIT volunteers (and now, its two staff members) couldn't easily dismiss it as the older generation just being out of touch.

The final reason for the break was more practical than ideological. Until then, the major funding for AIT had come from the county subcontract through the Asian Pacific AIDS Education Project. A/PLG had relied on the fiscal infrastructure of SSG and then APHCV as lead agencies. For the most part, Dean was able to handle AIT's administrative functions as the director of the Asian Pacific AIDS Education Project, with crucial assistance from Doug Chin, another A/PLG and AIT founding member and part of Dean's inner circle for more than a decade. A certified public accountant, Doug volunteered to keep books for the modest operation. With state funding, A/PLG became a primary contractor, and its internal controls and accounting system would come under much more intense scrutiny from the funder. The state expected a full-time fiscal manager, not a part-time volunteer. A/PLG didn't have that experience with such a funder, and Doug didn't want to shoulder the increasing responsibility. AIT, then, needed to shop for a fiscal sponsor.

They didn't have to go far. Dean had already had positive experience with SSG in the first funding cycle of the AIDS Education Project. SSG staff, Naomi and Paul, worked on the winning proposal to the state. In 1992, AIT members approached Herb Hatanaka, SSG's executive director, to see if his agency was willing to take them on. They met in the backroom at the Mayfair Hotel, close to SSG's office in Downtown LA. The AIT contingent included Dean, Ric, and Tak Yamamoto. "It was a smoky, dark room, very Yakuza style," Ric recalled. Their ask was simple and specific: Would SSG take on the AIDS Intervention Team as one of its divisions and handle all the contractual requirements from the state? Herb had something else in mind. He wanted to talk beyond the current state contract and "hammer out a long-term agreement."

"I told them, you could be problem-focused, like focusing on AIDS among APIs," Herb said. "However good and important that was, I was thinking about all the broader social issues that they were dealing with in their community, like health or mental health. As I saw it, nobody else was going to take those issues on." SSG's flagship divisions at the time were mental health-focused, and the agency would grow exponentially in the 2000s with the influx of public investment in mental and behavioral health in California. Herb saw how AIT could fit into his bigger picture for SSG, and SSG, in turn, would help them address these issues in the LGBTQ Asian American community. Herb knew SSG was "pretty strong as an organization at both the county and federal level. They could lean on SSG's credibility." In our interview, Herb easily rattled off three county supervisors at the time with whom he had a good relationship (including one who wasn't so friendly to the AIDS cause). Three out of the five supervisors made a majority, and that could help AIT's aspiring advocacy. The group was a little fearful that AIT would be swallowed under a bigger agency, but Herb assured them that the existing core leadership was what gave the project "that strong identity." He had no interest in taking over their project. In fact, he wouldn't be interested in helping them unless they agreed to continue steering the course. The strength of SSG, he told them, was to give grassroots leaders like them the infrastructure to succeed. He knew better than to mess with the leadership. As far as he was concerned, it was a win-win.

Herb's organizational approach convinced Ric and others that SSG was not just a good choice, but also the only viable one. Even in his early activism, Ric had heard mainstream AIDS service organization dismiss the idea of an agency addressing AIDS in the Asian American community. "A lot of people were baffled as to why we even had an API-specific organization," he remembered. "There were a lot of naysayers. They'd say, 'Oh, why do you guys even exist? They [APIs with HIV] can just come to us.'" These "naysayers" predicted that an organization like AIT couldn't be competitive for funding. And there Herb was that day, telling them the opposite: don't just focus on AIDS as a single issue; don't limit yourselves, think bigger. It was music to Ric's ears.

"The way he described his philosophy, I just saw this very strong, together, leader that could mentor us and help us get to the next level," Ric said. "I felt safe with him. And I trusted him."

Dean had already worked with SSG. Its infrastructure and experience with public funding all went into Dean's calculations prior to the meeting. There were other agencies with strong infrastructure that were interested in getting AIDS funding. What made a unique difference for Dean was the comfort level that Ric talked about. "[Herb] gave me the impression that he was not homophobic," Dean said. "I knew agencies who said they were not homophobic but turned out to have biases in their staff or board. Herb gave me the best feeling that he could abide by our goals and issues." That day, he was reassured that AIT would retain its independence it needed to grow.

Now, they could split with A/PLG without worrying about being homeless.

The A/PLG steering committee scheduled a meeting in June 1992 to discuss Dean's proposal to separate AIT from A/PLG. Some of the AIT members, including Ric, were in attendance. Once again, Sally and Terry played an instrumental role in this next phase of AIT development. They were asked to mediate between A/PLG and AIT to facilitate the separation. Though it was clear that the association was no longer sustainable for either side, the success and amicability of the conversation was by no means guaranteed. "The older guards, like Dean, who had a long-time affiliation with A/PLG, wanted to remain amiable," Sally recalled. They wanted a more conflict-averse approach so that they could preserve the relationship while figuring out a different arrangement. The younger people, according to Sally, were more idealistic and maybe impatient. They were dreaming big and ready to pull away. "They wanted to own their own building or become a one-stop shop for the community, sort of an API version of AIDS Project Los Angeles. Some of the older people were rolling their eyes. We had to do some reality testing with them." As cofacilitators, Sally and Terry had to walk a fine line among the factions. Ric remembered Sally and Terry being "academic" in their approach and setting ground rules about how they should talk, about active listening, about being appropriate, but people on all sides had been holding back what they wanted to say to each other. The confrontation was as inevitable as the evening tides that no painstakingly careful facilitation plan could stem.

"It was ugly," Ric said of that meeting. "But in an Asian ugly way. People weren't screaming or hollering at each other. The tension was in the air. You could cut it with a knife. We all knew this was a turning point. Let me tell you this—all the White boys on their side were doing all the talking. They were doing all the negotiations for an API organization. The Asian guys were sitting there passively and saying nothing." It was the kind of dynamic that Ric thought would be toxic to the AIDS work. "That's when we knew we weren't only fighting on the outside. We were also fighting internally for change."

At issue was more than just the matter of spinoff. AIT already had an operating budget larger than what A/PLG was able to raise through its membership dues and fundraising events. The AIT side contended that these public dollars belonged to the community and that they needed to go with AIT to SSG. With steadily bigger contracts, A/PLG leaders couldn't deny that this was an important community issue anymore, even if they had no intention or know-how to address it. They wouldn't be able to keep the funds if they couldn't do the work. People had one last chance to air what they had been meaning to say. With Doug Chin's careful accounting of AIT finances, the amount of transfer was unassailable. After all that was said and done, the two sides agreed to separate.

The history of an AIDS project separating from its more socially oriented LGBTQ parent organization was not unique to AIT. Bienestar, now one of the largest AIDS service organizations in LA, began modestly in 1985 as an HIV educational committee of Gay and Lesbian Latinos Unidos, or GLLU, founded in 1981. Like AIT at A/PLG, Bienestar at first provided support exclusively to GLLU members who became HIV positive. Oscar de la O, its founding director, recalled a particular GLLU member falling ill from HIV. He said, "I reached out to him, and he didn't even want to see me. For the first two, three months, I took him food and left it outside his door." The member rebuffed Oscar's offer to clean his house, and Oscar just left clean sheets for him so he could at least change his bed. Also like AIT, Bienestar's efforts were snubbed from the very beginning by many gay men in their parent organization. "The women, the lesbians of GLLU, were extremely supportive, but there was resistance from the men," Oscar said. "At least the ones in leadership roles felt that the HIV work would overshadow GLLU." According to Oscar, the GLLU leadership saw the Bienestar volunteers "as an extension of what they could do for GLLU." Oscar had to insist that they "were there to focus on HIV work, not to be putting out newsletters or other work for GLLU." Like Dean, Oscar attributed this resistance to internalized stigma. In 1991, Bienestar separated from GLLU and became its own nonprofit organization. At least for these two organizations in LGBTQ communities of color in LA, the antagonists in their first chapter were often their own kin.

AIT followed Bienestar's suit closely. In 1992, in a matter of months of receiving the state's contract and the meeting at Mayfair Hotel, AIT migrated to SSG and changed its name to the Asian Pacific AIDS Intervention Team, or APAIT. Dean concurrently held the position of paid full-time director of Asian Pacific AIDS Education Project and volunteer APAIT division director, until he could find a replacement for the former. Once again, he drew from AIT's pool of young activists and recruited Eric Reyes. Eric had been a volunteer when he was an urban planning graduate student at UCLA. After he graduated, Eric wasn't sure he wanted to pursue a doctorate program right away, and his activism with Colors United primed him to consider HIV/AIDS as the defining issue around which to organize the broader LGBTQ Asian American community. Dean appreciated Eric's academic approach; it was an appreciation that would guide their interactions in the subsequent years. When he asked Eric to take over, Eric said yes.

As Dean predicted, with the funding paradigm shift to targeted outreach and behavioral modification, the Asian Pacific AIDS Education Project's approach of general outreach eventually fell out of favor. Many organizations in the partnership stopped doing AIDS work by the late 1990s, while at least one, SIPA, successfully sought county funding for its targeted outreach in the Filipino American community. Under Kazue Shibata's leadership, APHCV expanded and took off in a new direction. By 1997, APHCV had moved out of the Chinatown Annex and opened what would be the first of several community health centers across LA.

CHAPTER 6

School of Fish

BY THE TIME THE DUST SETTLED AND THE ASIAN PACIFIC AIDS
Intervention Team (APAIT) emerged in 1992, Los Angeles had
developed an AIDS industry that had its own hierarchy, with people of
color on the bottom rung, as many critics contended. In 1987, LA County
established its commission on AIDS to, in the words of county supervisor
Ed Edelman, "look at the financial aspect of the County AIDS related
programs and services and determine the adequacy of resources allocation and the effectiveness in the utilization of these services."[1] It made
recommendations to the county on how much to fund different service
categories (like hospice care and outreach). The commission vetted policies on partner notification, a medical ward specifically for AIDS
patients, and bathhouse closure. They even asked the county to take positions against another AIDS quarantine ballot initiative in California in
1988 (which, like its predecessor two years before, also failed) and state
legislation that would have denied health insurance to people with HIV.

A few months after its formation in August 1987, the commission listened to a presentation by Dr. Caswell A. Evans, from the county's
Department of Health Services, on the gaps and needs in AIDS education. Dr. Evans suggested that there was "substantial behavior modification" in the gay population and concluded that the safer sex message had
been effectively suffused in that community—for the most part. He cau-
tioned that "concern should still be expressed about the spread of the
virus around the periphery of the Gay community." By "periphery,"

Dr. Evans meant "men who have sex with other men but who do not identify themselves as homosexual or gay, and young men perhaps experimenting with that lifestyle." He went on to highlight that "the risk for exposure and development of AIDS among minorities is substantial."[2]

The epidemiological data would bear out what Dr. Evans had predicted in late 1987. According to the AIDS Monthly Surveillance Report, non-Hispanic Whites accounted for 69 percent of people with AIDS in LA County before 1988 but dropped to 60 percent in 1988 and to 54 percent in 1991. Black and Brown people had a reverse trendline. African Americans accounted for 14 percent of people with AIDS before 1988, but rose to 19 percent in 1988. That number did stabilize in the next few years. For Latinos, the percentage went from 15 percent before 1988 to 20 percent in 1988 and 26 percent in 1991.

The advocates who toiled in communities of color had already known that. Almost as soon as the LA County AIDS Commission was established, they lobbied it to expand and diversify its membership. At its first meeting in 1987, agency members on the AIDS commission included major players in the primary care safety net for the county, such as Hospital Council of Southern California and Los Angeles County Medical Association, as well as representatives from federal agencies, such as the Centers for Disease Control and Prevention and the US surgeon general. The commission also included two mainstream AIDS service providers, AIDS Project Los Angeles (APLA) and the Gay and Lesbian Community Services Center (GLCSC). In February 1988, commissioner Alvin Ransom attended a panel organized by the local NAACP chapter. Soon after, Rabbi Allen I. Freehling, who chaired the commission, wrote a memo to the commission, acknowledging that Ransom was asked to deliver a message from the Black community. The memo read, "If the AIDS Commission intends to properly reflect Black community input, it must add additional representatives. Notably missing are (1) representation from the Minority AIDS Project and (2) professional representation such as a physician member of the Charles R. Drew Medical Society."[3] The request was a clear rebuke to the commission membership's lack of diversity and its inability to address the needs of the Black community, or communities of color in general.

APLA, in particular, was becoming the behemoth that behemoths often are—very necessary and a little evil in the eyes of some; Joël Tan described it as "both resources and assholes at the same time." In 1982, a group that would become the APLA founders met with representatives from the Kaposi's Sarcoma Foundation from San Francisco (now the San Francisco AIDS Foundation) to learn about the disease that was just beginning to plague that city. After the meeting, the LA group urgently established a hotline to answer questions that would surely follow as rumors about the epidemic spread. What began as a modest volunteer operation serving five clients in early 1983 quickly became a bona fide nonprofit organization, with more than a hundred clients by the end of that year (that number would double in another six months). By the mid-1980s, Sally Jue, who was working at APLA at the time, recalled that the agency received not one but three big demonstration grants from the Health Resources and Services Administration, a federal agency, to provide mental health services and housing. Very few cities were getting any federal AIDS funding at all. With this influx, APLA spun off in two additional locations.

As early as 1983, according to an *LA Weekly* article by writer and activist Doug Sadownick, some LGBTQ community leaders, "angered by what they saw as APLA's emerging bureaucracy, founded Aid for AIDS to offer money directly to needy PWAs [People with AIDS]." Sadownick went on: "That same year, the LA Shanti Foundation emerged to deal with the emotional grief surrounding AIDS, which APLA didn't handle. Groups like Being Alive [which was run by PWAs for PWAs] were founded to watch AIDS agencies they had felt had grown too large to minister to PWAs effectively."[4]

And these were just the complaints from the White gay community.

APLA and the mainstream AIDS service organizations in the 1980s rarely ventured out of the gay strongholds in LA, and if you were a gay man of color who didn't work, live, or play in West Hollywood or Silverlake, these services were not going to touch you. If the critics were kind, this just mirrored the existing racial segregation in the gay community. Phill Wilson, a longtime AIDS activist in the Black community, explained it this way:

> In the early days, I do not believe there was malicious neglect. All folks were doing was trying to save themselves and their friends. [The virus] was like an army of mad men with machine guns just running

through all of our communities, just shooting, shooting, shooting and all people were trying to do was just not die. What AIDS showed is that if you were White, your friends were White, or that so few White gay men had real relationships with men of color. If people organized out of their telephone books, which is what they did, there were so few people of color in those telephone books.

This benign neglect was a reflection of "the inherent, embedded racism in the gay community." He continued, "Now, it wasn't that when Black or Latino or Asian people would go there, they would be turned away. But there was no aggressive acknowledgment that the epidemic was even impacting us. No notion around cultural competency or the need to develop program that were specific and explicit. It just wasn't part of their consciousness. All of our activism was in response to that lack."

Oscar de la O at Bienestar remembered that the executive director of APLA took umbrage at his characterization of APLA's relationship with communities of color as one of "neglect." In moments of conciliation, Oscar would sometimes switch to the concept of "cultural competence." That is, it wasn't that mainstream gay providers didn't want to acknowledge or serve people of color; it was more that they didn't know how to. The concept was consistent with the advocacy by grassroots organizations in communities of color to justify their existence and worthiness for funding to those policymakers who were still acclimating to the idea that the gay community could be racist.

Initially, people stayed in their lanes. "They [the mainstream AIDS service organizations] didn't try to work with us, but I wouldn't say they resisted our efforts," Phill recalled. "They could say, 'Well, if Bienestar is treating Latinos and APAIT is treating Asians and the Minority AIDS Project is treating Black people, we don't have to worry about it.' They'd think it's covered." The smaller and newer organizations serving communities of color hadn't had a track record in competing for funding to provide direct services to people with AIDS and didn't represent a threat. Instead, the mainstream organizations used these smaller groups as a pass to doing outreach outside of the White gay community.

For their part, activists of color focused on strengthening their own capacity. "We weren't that interested in partnership," Phill continued, "especially with APLA, because we understood that it was really important for us to build institutions in our communities to take care of ourselves. The history of colonialism, patriarchy, and tokenism had not served us well." Bigger organizations might have more resources, but leaders like Phill, Oscar, and Dean did not want to make a habit of relying on them.

That was the state of the AIDS industry during those early years of the LA County AIDS Commission. As the memo by the commission chair, Rabbi Freehling, hinted, activists of color had to fight their way to find a place at the table. In 1988, about a year after its formation, the AIDS commission, along with the LA County Commission on Human Relations, cosponsored a hearing on the impact of AIDS on people of color. Reverend Carl Bean from the Minority AIDS Project spoke on the racial inequity of AIDS funding distribution. Psychologist Terry Gock, who chaired the HIV/AIDS task force at APPCON, talked about how AIDS affected the Asian population and advocated for the need for culturally and linguistically sensitive services in a community that encompassed almost twenty different cultural traditions and even more languages and dialects.

The hearing resulted in a report, in which Terry continued to hit on other key advocacy points that Asian American AIDS activists would repeat for years to come. He referenced the "alarming" increase in the number of Asians with AIDS in LA, based on epidemiological data that had disaggregated Asians from the "Other" category only recently. In addition to the cultural and linguistic barriers, Terry discussed the Asian American community's "strong tendency to deny that AIDS is a concern for their population." Albert Ogle, from All Saints Episcopal Church in Pasadena, wrote about the concentration of AIDS-related services in traditional gay venues because APLA, the major recipient of federal and state funding at the time, "chose to operate centralized programs." This, argued Ogle, left out neighborhoods and ethnic or racial groups that desperately needed these services.

In response, the commission began to invite experts to discuss issues that were specific to people with AIDS in minority communities, such as the intersection between undocumented immigration and HIV status.

In February 1990, J Craig Fong, a public interest attorney, testified before the AIDS commission on federal immigration policy. At the time, J was working for the Los Angeles County Bar Association, as the assistant director of its Immigration Project. His comments touched on how current immigration policies impacted immigrants with HIV primarily in the Latino community. According to the commission minutes,

> Mr. Fong stated that the immigrants to the US are the only civilian non-criminal population in the US that are subject to universal testing. This population is excludable from the US and subject to deportation if they test seropositive. This also affects the amnesty population with primary impact on the Hispanic community. . . . The Hispanic community is very susceptible to fear. Mr. Fong stated that LA is the highest amnesty impact area and is one of the top three impact areas for all immigrants to come into the US. He would like to see an educational outreach program geared toward the immigrant population. He stressed that this population is very sensitive to anything that will affect immigration status. They are a very receptive educable population.

J was born in the mid-1950s in the Bay Area and had worked in law firms in both San Francisco and Chicago before relocating to LA in 1985 to direct an immigration project for a civil rights advocacy organization in the Asian American community. How did someone like J end up testifying in front of an official AIDS commission about the needs of the Latino community?

In 1986, shortly after he had started his job in LA, President Ronald Reagan signed an immigration reform bill that offered amnesty to undocumented immigrants who had entered the US before 1982. Despite some fears that this might be a trap to lure these immigrants, millions of them came forward and sought help applying for a green card. The organization J was working for had staff members who were fluent in multiple Asian languages, and also Spanish, so his team was helping some immigrants from Mexico and Latin America in this process. Around the same time, federal AIDS policy began to target immigrants and even tourists, with HIV. In 1987, Congress passed what was known as the Helms Amendment (named after the North Carolina Republican senator Jesse Helms) to include HIV on a list of "excludable conditions" to keep people with HIV out of the country. This HIV ban was what J was referring to in his testimony to the AIDS commission. Interestingly enough, while immigration was becoming generally more liberal in the mid-1980s under the conservative Reagan administration, it was moving in the opposite direction for immigrants with HIV. In fact, if they had come forward to ask for amnesty, their HIV status might be revealed, which would likely lead to their deportation.

"Not a lot of people paid attention to that," J said, because immigrants with HIV constituted a fraction of those seeking amnesty. The intersection between HIV and immigration was often lost on policymakers and activists who focused on one or the other. Even if AIDS advocates in the immigrant communities wanted to do something, they didn't have the legal expertise or connections to make their voices heard, and legal advocates, overwhelmed by the amnesty push, didn't make HIV a priority. A Chinese American gay man and a son of immigrants, J's personal and professional identities straddled this intersection and led him to become a unique and necessary voice in the HIV discourse for immigrants.

As he began to see people who came in "with no alternative for them," J teamed up with attorneys in San Francisco, Chicago, and Boston "to create a mechanism that allowed people who had HIV who were applying for amnesty to get a waiver in order to get that green card." "Of course, the word got out," he recalled, "not just for Asian Americans, but anybody who was HIV positive, because nobody else would touch them. The attorneys in LA really didn't understand AIDS at that point, not until, I would say, the middle to late '90s. Before that, it was all superstition."

Meanwhile, management at his agency felt that AIDS fell outside their purview and discouraged J from taking on these cases. "It was hard enough working with undocumented immigrants," J said. "There were still a lot of people who didn't like foreigners." His supervisor warned, "Don't spend too much time on this. [AIDS is] just not an Asian problem." J didn't think his supervisor was homophobic, but rather that he buckled under the fear of reprisals from donors, from community at large, or from the general public, who would associate the organization with such a stigmatized population. Though furious, J persisted.

As the management expected, the project drew national attention—but it was mostly positive recognition. "Everywhere west of the Mississippi, people were calling us," J said. "My work connected me with all kinds of gay and lesbian organizations nationwide. Even gay men and lesbians who didn't have HIV would come to us because they realized we were gay and lesbian friendly. They could come to us for their amnesty and immigration problems because they wouldn't feel like they were being judged by their immigration attorney." The agency was thrust onto the national stage not because of any of its bread-and-butter, Asian-American-focused projects, but precisely because it was taking up an issue—AIDS—that not many civil or immigrant rights organizations would come near at the time. Their worst fears were not realized, and J noted that years later, the same supervisor who had discouraged him became a strong ally of gay and lesbian causes, including same-sex marriage.

The immigration project motivated J to "connect with APIs who were dealing with AIDS and APIs dealing with gay and lesbian issues." He remembered one undocumented client from 1987 whose family was so ashamed of him that they refused to cooperate with J. When the client fell ill, the family took him home to Monterey Park, and J's access to the client became even more restricted. "The family kept him in the garage," He said. "They fed him on paper plates and with plastic knives and forks. They never let him see his friends. I never got a chance to finish his case. I never legalized him."

J also connected this tragedy to his close friend who died of AIDS around the same time:

> He was Chinese Cuban. We were in law school together. He was my partner in crime, my best bar buddy, the person that I gossiped and shared adventures with. But when he got sick enough, his family came and took him back to Florida. . . . His boyfriend couldn't even get in touch with him. I actually felt. . . . For anybody who knows me, I guess this sounds unusual, but I felt tongue-tied. How do I say to the family, "Look, he's dying. How can I help?" I confess that I didn't have a lot of vocabulary to reach out to them and say, "He still needs to be with his community. He still needs his friends around him." I'm somewhat ashamed that I wasn't strong enough to figure out what to do. And then he was gone. There are still days when I think I should have done more. . . . I should have been somehow magically more connected with medicine and with community groups. I kicked myself because I wasn't.

Both his bar buddy and his clients made clear for J the need for more concerted outreach efforts to find people in immigrant communities who needed help, because they weren't always going to come seek it. He also recognized that he couldn't do it alone. Though he was a legal expert, he needed to come with someone who had the vocabulary that he lacked, someone with more resources to offer, like social support, counseling, or information about treatments. J put out feelers and found Daniel Lara, who was working at APLA at the time. Through Lara, J connected with Bienestar. He had an idea for outreach that he wanted tested. He called his approach "a bait and switch." J explained:

> We would do a presentation on immigration. Nice and safe. We used it as a hook to bring in the Latinos. Ironically immigration was non-threatening because we were not talking about sex and death. We started with green cards. We didn't start with AIDS or homosexuality. Then we'd say, "By the way, in order to get your green card, you're going to need to take an AIDS test. You need to know your status before you walk over to immigration and apply for your green card. You need to know before the government knows."

Then his partners would "slip in information about AIDS."

Often, J had to present the immigration information in Spanish because they couldn't find enough Spanish-speaking attorneys comfortable enough to "reach over that divide and talk about AIDS." He said, "They saw some Chinese guy walking into a Mexican or Latino church, and they looked at me like, 'Who's this guy?' The community groups let me in as a Chinese American man. They said, 'You know what? Your Spanish is a little funny, but we trust you.'"

J tested out this bait-and-switch strategy in the Latino community first before he made connections with Dean and others to replicate it in the Asian American community. He recalled making several presentations to LGBTQ Asian American organizations, including Asian/Pacific Lesbians and Gays (A/PLG). Outwardly, A/PLG members gave him a cordial reception. It was only in private that some of the White A/PLG members approached J for help for their Asian friends or lovers. Some things still hadn't changed.

Over the years, Dean and his staff at APAIT would refer any clients who needed immigration help to J. He continued to be a resource for

APAIT and other agencies even after he left his public interest role in the nonprofit sector and moved into his private practice, where he took these cases on a pro-bono basis (the HIV immigration ban was finally lifted only in 2010). When Dean Goishi established a community advisory board at APAIT shortly after it migrated to Special Service for Groups (SSG), J was one of the first people he asked to serve.

As the director of the Asian Pacific AIDS Education Project, Dean also attended the commission meetings regularly to remind policymakers that Asians with HIV existed. He talked about some of their efforts and reiterated the same advocacy points that Terry had discussed at the 1988 hearing. In the early years of the epidemic, the biggest problem for Asian American AIDS advocates was that there was no data available; Asians were lumped with the "Other" category. When the AIDS incidence rate and other statistics became disaggregated around 1986 in LA County, things didn't become easier for the activists. Now, the number that was attached to the "Asian" category in the surveillance reports was very low compared to other racial groups, constituting around 1 to 2 percent of all HIV diagnoses annually. As Terry suggested, even when the number of diagnoses was almost doubling from one year to the next in the late eighties, this represented fewer than fifty new HIV cases in the Asian community—this during a period in which between 2,000 and 2,500 individuals per year were learning that they had contracted HIV. Funding allocations were tied to incidence rates in the respective community. Not having the numbers, the Asian community was vulnerable to being dismissed by policymakers. By this time, all the major and minor players were jockeying for positions in anticipation of bigger funding streams trickling from the federal government. Dean and other Asian American activists had much ground to cover in order to catch up.

It was at venues like the AIDS commission and other public hearings where early Asian American AIDS advocates like Terry and Dean learned to hone their arguments. These arguments fell into three categories, which Terry and Dean presented in varying combinations to suit the situation and the audience. First, the activists cast doubts on the low incidence rate in the Asian community and suggested that more Asians were HIV-positive than reported in official data. Second, regardless of incidence rate, activists argued for more prevention resources to be allocated to the Asian community. Third, they explained that the linguistic diversity in the Asian community required additional resources in order to serve especially the immigrant populations.

For the first argument, activists offered many explanations on why the HIV-incidence rate was underreported. A number of scientific studies showed that Asians tended to seek medical help later than other communities, not just for HIV, but in general. Some studies have also shown that many immigrants would turn to traditional healers and medicine before they consulted a doctor. Most advocates resorted to a cultural explanation for this delay; that is, Asian cultural attitudes about health and disease didn't encourage people to get tested or turn to doctors until the conditions became so debilitating that they prevented them from performing their work or other obligations. With AIDS, cultural stigma made it even more daunting for those who knew they were at risk to find out about their status. AIDS stigma existed in all communities, but because the Asian community—as all immigrant communities—was so tightly knit, the stigma took on a unique cultural dimension. As Sally Jue explained, the interdependence of family members meant that everyone in a household was expected to contribute to its long-term economic survival. For younger people, that could mean educational advancement that was denied to many of their immigrant parents. She said, "If you're from a middle- or lower-class background, or if you've got immigrant parents who have that expectation of you, you're probably less likely to do something that could derail that, to cause you to have a serious rift with your family." Many gay men in these immigrant households would not only have to hide their sexuality for the sake of harmony, but also not seek help even when they suspected to have contracted the virus, if that help exposed them and threatened that harmony.

In a public testimony to the commission in 1995, APAIT staff Tracy Nako stated:

> In my experience working with HIV+ APIs, shame, silence, and
> cultural denial are common factors which delay people from getting
> tested early. As a result, most of the clients we see have had PCP
> [pneumocystis pneumonia] and are AIDS diagnosed with very low
> T-cells. . . . The fear [of disclosure] is so great that [a client] may

hesitate to access any services. . . . He was taught that as a man, an Asian man, he must solve his problems alone. To air them out is a sign of weakness and there is a loss of face or shame. . . . This ultimately leads to isolation and sometimes depression.[5]

Tracy's testimony was fairly typical. The cultural explanation seemed to be more prevalent than other arguments, perhaps because cultural defi-cits were an easier pill for policymakers to swallow than any call for fun-damental systemic changes. Asian American AIDS advocates could still score points for why their services were necessary, without alienating the audience.

Fewer advocates and researchers promoted more structural explana-tions for underreporting and delayed care, citing poverty, immigration sta-tus, the lack of health insurance for many immigrants or the lack of cultural and linguistically competent care in mainstream medical establishments. Because of these barriers in HIV, as in other diseases like cancer, research confirmed, Asians were diagnosed later, when the symptoms became more severe. The underreporting in HIV incidence rate, argued the advocates, was just the tip of a much bigger but hidden health crisis. This argument worked well to suggest the importance of outreach and education to encourage people in the Asian American community to get tested for HIV so that they could become aware of the risks they posed to themselves and others with whom they might have unsafe sex or share needles.

Whether cultural or structural, these arguments for underreporting were important because AIDS funding was tied to the infection rate in specific communities. Early advocates came up with the second argu-ment to reframe the official data and appeal to policymakers for more prevention dollars. If the AIDS incidence rate was indeed as low as the official epidemiological data suggested, advocates argued for more out-reach and education to keep the disease from infiltrating and spreading into the community. But if there were more Asians living with HIV who were not coming forward, as the underreporting arguments suggested, the community needed to find them and convince them to get tested and access health services that they were eligible for. To convince people to come out, the public health message needed to reduce AIDS stigma in the Asian American community. Either way, advocates tried to educate policymakers why the Asian American community "had a right to prevention resources." "APAIT and our [APPCON HIV Task Force] had to convince [policymakers] that here was a good opportunity to stop [HIV] from spreading [in the Asian American community]," Terry Gock said. "However, selling prevention is very hard. We have to just keep hammering it." Sally remembered pleading at a HIV conference, "The goal of prevention is to prevent people from getting sick. So how many of us have to die before we are deemed worthy of prevention funds?"

When policymakers conceded any of these arguments, early advocates then used the third argument to squeeze a little more resource from them: the linguistic diversity of the Asian American community (or communities, really). To be able to reach and serve those who were linguistically isolated and had the least access to both health care and prevention messages, providers would need additional translation and interpretation services and a multilingual staff with enough cultural capital to penetrate all these separate immigrant communities that might not share a sense of pan-ethnic Asian identity.

In fact, translation and interpretation services were among the early concessions from the county in addressing the AIDS epidemic in the Asian American community. In 1991, the Asian Pacific AIDS Education Project received a modest grant from the county to provide translation services. In 1993, according to Naomi Kageyama, the county dedicated $20,000, "leftover" from some funding mechanism, for SSG to help limited English proficient (LEP) Asians living with HIV to access services—a stopgap alternative to holding mainstream providers accountable to serve this population. The funding was meant to placate community advocates. (To be fair, no other health programs in the county health department had been as welcoming to language interpretation as the Office of AIDS Programs and Policy.) With this allocation, SSG started a parallel program to APAIT called Pacific Asian Language Services (PALS). In addition to her development responsibilities at SSG, Naomi was tasked to operate and grow PALS as its program director. PALS would go on to train cadres of multilingual interpreters in any medical setting—not only for HIV/AIDS—and to hold county facilities and private hospitals accountable for complying with federal laws around language access for LEP patients. But its origins had everything to do with AIDS advocacy—just one example of how AIDS transformed the broader health delivery system.

People who knew and worked with Dean would invariably describe him as soft-spoken. He himself shunned the activist label and would only say that he was an introvert unwittingly being thrusted under the public spotlight. Yet early on, he knew that in the positions he held at the AIDS Education Project and later at APAIT, he had to get in front of the policymakers and do many things outside of his comfort zone. "If you're not sitting at the table, you're not going to be heard. If you're not heard, you miss out," he said. From talking with and watching other AIDS activists, Dean learned that he needed to "yell to not be left out." He learned public speaking by speaking publicly. The lessons were "fast and steep"; spaces like the AIDS commission were his school. He drummed his points about Asian American community needs over and over again, even when his targets had heard them before. Years later, Dean said that if he were given an opportunity to talk about Asians and AIDS in public, "you'd have to drag me off the stage." To me, Dean was a perfect illustration of how leaders are made, not born. They are people who become extraordinary because they answer the call for a broader good. And it takes all types and personalities.

Dean and other Asian American AIDS activists didn't fight these advocacy battles alone. Quite the contrary. Their success was a testament to multiracial organizing among communities of color in LA, at a time when strife among African Americans, Latinos, and Asians took up a lot more oxygen in our airwaves than cooperation did. These flames erupted most spectacularly in the 1992 LA uprising that followed the acquittal of four LAPD officers who were caught beating Black motorist Rodney King. In AIDS advocacy, the LGBTQ communities of color presented a united front, mostly through the Gay Men of Color Consortium (GMOCC).

GMOCC was a coalition that included Bienestar, Black and White Men Together, Minority AIDS Project, and Teatro VIVA. A/PLG was a member until AIT split off in 1992. Shortly after that, APAIT officially joined the consortium. GMOCC first came together about the same time the AIDS commission was established. Phill Wilson was a leader with Black and White Men Together then. He had moved to LA in 1982 from Chicago, where he grew up in a housing project in the south side—"as far south as you could go in Chicago and still be in the city limits." He said,

"I actually didn't even meet a real live White person until I was five." The leaders in his organization as well as in the Gay and Lesbian Latinos Unidos (GLLU) and A/PLG, all membership organizations with more of a social mission "were struggling in how they were going to respond to AIDS" in their respective community. Even before these organizations started doing AIDS work, they were supporting each other's events. The 1986 AIDS quarantine initiative further crystallized the need to act politically. "The way we fought that initiative actually forged the bonds that would later on create the foundation for the coalition of people of color here in Los Angeles," Phill said. He remembered how vocal the Asian American community was in drawing the parallels between the quarantine of people with AIDS and the Japanese American concentration camps during World War II. The tenor of the protests by people of color was very different from the gay White mainstream. In his *LA Weekly* article, AIDS activist Doug Sadownick wrote, "Stop the AIDS Quarantine [led by Phill and his partner Chris Brownlie] organized a torchlight march on LaRouche's headquarters that the tame 'No on 64' leaders did everything in their power to prevent. Leaders called it 'too angry, too gay.'" These White gay leaders, whom Sadownick described as "corporate westsiders," wanted to "fight the proposition on issues of cost-effectiveness, not gay rights," and they were "not interested in building a Rainbow-style coalition of gays, Latinos, and blacks."[6]

White exclusion helped the "angry" queer communities of color coalesce. The triumvirate of A/PLG, Black and White Men Together, and GLLU already had a history of working together. Phill said, "In part because Oscar [de la O] and Dean and I were friends from our work mobilizing LGBT people of color, from the very, very beginning, we just understood there was a need to work together. I'm not even positive that there was much a discussion."

According to Phill, GMOCC existed for three purposes: sharing best practices, increasing the visibility of gay men of color, and collective advocacy. He said that they were "just figuring out a way so that there was funding that explicitly targeted men of color and then, secondly, that there were eligibility criteria in place to increase the competitiveness for organizations that were rooted in those communities." GMOCC became a vessel through which these agencies could apply for and receive grants that they would otherwise be unable to compete for on their own. Their funding revolved around joint efforts in social marketing and promotion of services to gay men of color, but it was perhaps in collective advocacy where GMOCC had the most impact.

In those initial years, GMOCC members were small fish in a big pond, each unable to effect a noticeable ripple on their own. Even with data showing incidence rates rising faster among people of color than the White gay population, the assumption among policymakers or even LGBTQ media was to invest in organizations with a larger infrastructure than these upstart organizations in communities of color, with the wishful thinking that these bigger organizations, like APLA, would eventually figure out how to diversify their client populations and the staff who served them. The message that these bigger mainstream agencies were not the most proficient in targeting gay men of color "had to be constantly repeated at the proposal review sessions," said Dean. "Most of the reviewers were not always involved in the community here in LA, and so they thought, 'Well, give it to APLA because they were the biggest and they probably were the best and most successful.' Maybe in Hollywood or West Hollywood, but not in East LA, South Central, or any of the Asian Towns." Dean and others remembered instances well into the 1990s where the bigger agencies would receive huge public contracts to serve people of color and come to the GMOCC members only later, offering paltry subcontracts in exchange for help to get into the very communities that these bigger agencies had written into their proposals.

Shawn Griffin cited an incendiary article in 1991 about the AIDS service landscape in LA, published in *Edge*, a since-defunct weekly in the LGBTQ community. Shawn, an African American, was a member of the Gay and Lesbian Alliance Against Defamation (GLAAD) at the time, an organization that monitors media representation of LGBTQ people. He said, "The article said there was no need for community-specific HIV and AIDS services, that it should be one organization, APLA, serving everybody." The article went on to argue that these organizations were "duplicative." Some people in communities of color "took offense to that" and took their complaints to GLAAD. GLAAD was accustomed to holding mainstream media accountable for realistic portrayals of the LGBTQ community. But this complaint was directed at one of the community's own media outlets about racial insensitivity. GLAAD turned to Shawn to help put together a delegation to meet with the editors at *Edge*. Shawn found Ric Parish, who introduced him to Crispin Rosas, the executive director of GMOCC. Together, GLAAD and GMOCC members expressed their indignation to the editors. As a result, *Edge* agreed to publish a counterpoint, which Shawn and another GLAAD member cowrote, with a sidebar that listed all the AIDS service organizations in communities of color. A year later, Rosas hired Shawn to be his assistant at GMOCC, and Shawn succeeded him as the executive director in 1993.

On the surface, things seemed cordial between the big and small fish. However, when the pond got bigger, things began to change, especially with the demographic shifts in HIV incidence. Shawn said, "When the face of the disease changed, that's when these [mainstream] agencies started applying for money for gay men of color. Sometimes it worked out well. Sometimes it didn't." For instance, APLA had tried to make themselves relevant to non-White communities, sometimes by poaching people of color who had risen up through the ranks in the smaller AIDS service organizations in those communities, according to Oscar. Those early efforts smacked of tokenism. In the mid-1980s, Arturo Olivas, project director at Cara a Cara, a Latino AIDS outreach project, organized a protest at a public hearing where APLA was about to receive a $2.2 million grant, criticizing the bigger agency for ignoring the epidemic in the Latino community. In response, APLA hired Daniel Lara as a health educator. Lara was a rising star in the Latino AIDS movement. After he passed away of AIDS, the city named an HIV clinic after him. After a brief stint at APLA, however, Lara conceded "that he was placed at APLA as a stooge to undercut Olivas's efforts, not to effect any lasting change." Frustrated that APLA "had abandoned minorities," Lara resigned.

GMOCC members knew they had to stick together through these ruses. Recalling those early years in the AIDS commission, Oscar said that "there were a lot of back room deals and people calling for a break so that they would go and talk. That's when we started to come to the meetings saying, 'We're being left out.'" The idea of GMOCC took root at these meetings, Oscar added, to the point where "everyone knew not to propose something unless they were also talking about men of color."

I interviewed Dean (APAIT), Oscar (Bienestar), and Phill (Black and White Men Together, among many hats he would wear both locally and nationally later) separately. All three used the same phrase—"We had each other's back"—to describe their fellowship. The colloquialism is common enough, but they also gave the same detail to illustrate what they meant: if one of them was not in a room, he wouldn't be worried. He knew the other two would advocate for his community as if he were there himself.

"None of us ever had to say, 'I'm not getting enough,'" Oscar recalled. "We knew we were not going to take more than what we needed to ensure we had enough for everybody. That comes from respecting and knowing other communities." Shawn made a similar observation, especially about APAIT: "APAIT recognized the services that were needed in the API community. At the same time, there were several times [at the commission] when they would take to the mic and say, 'As much as we need this money for our community, we think it will be better served if the money went to another community.' They didn't make it always all about them. APAIT really set the example."

If the bigger mainstream agencies were willing to play with these smaller organizations, it was because GMOCC made it a "political practicality." Oscar said, "They saw that we [GMOCC] had come together, that we spoke one after the other and talked about the same needs. We would show up with thirty or forty people to give testimonials at a meeting. That showed our strength in front of the council members."

For the most part, GMOCC member agencies refused to be divided and conquered and survived any superficial efforts of tokenism. In 1990, testifying on the county's three-year HIV strategic plan, Gilberto Gerald, executive director of Minority AIDS Project (MAP), discussed how to balance the needs of diverse communities. The biggest GMOCC member at the time, MAP didn't have a large base of Asian American clients. Nevertheless, Gerald testified that "for other ethnic groups, such as the Asian communities, HIV-positive clients struggle with the issue of disclosure and what impact it may have on their family in regards to family status in the community. Consequently, some individuals will opt not to seek treatment and thus progress rapidly to AIDS and die a very isolated death." In other words, Gerald was making the same argument that Dean and other Asian American AIDS activists were making in their advocacy. At a time when epidemiological data didn't do any favors to the Asian population funding wise, it would've been so easy for the Black and Latino communities to shut them out. The numbers were increasingly on their side. But the opposite happened: there was trust, cooperation, and solidarity. That was when GMOCC was at its strongest, and member agencies like Bienestar and APAIT started to expand as a result of being part of it.

GMOCC was getting stronger at the right moment. The early 1990s were a watershed era for federal AIDS funding. In 1990, Congress passed the Ryan White Comprehensive AIDS Resources Emergency (CARE) Act. Before that, there had been brief moments when the American public would recognize the disease, like in 1985 when actor Rock Hudson, the quintessential American leading man from decades past, announced that he was afflicted with AIDS. Other than that, fighting AIDS was mostly a community-driven affair. AIDS service organizations toiled and cared for those high-risk populations that had been obscured from the public, and AIDS activists, like those from ACT UP, fought the government's indifference and kept AIDS in the national conversation. Their call for public investment in research, prevention, and treatment was met initially with modest concessions of federal funding. The Health Resources and Service Administration (HRSA), an agency under the Department of Health and Human Services, established AIDS service demonstration grants in 1986 that provided some relief, totaling a little over $15 million, to only four cities with high number of AIDS cases. Deemed "high-impact urban areas," they included LA, Miami, New York, and San Francisco. The following year, HRSA began the AIDS Drug Assistance Program to help those who otherwise couldn't afford the medication.

In 1987, a thirteen-year-old with HIV was thrust into the limelight. Hailing from Indiana, hardly an epicenter of the AIDS crisis, Ryan White had contracted HIV a few years before through a contaminated blood product that was used to treat his hemophilia. Many parents, school officials, and teachers in White's community tried to keep him out of school. Confrontations in and out of courts were played out for months in the nightly news. Even after it was resolved, White and his mother continued to speak publicly about AIDS paranoia and discrimination. White eventually died in 1990, outliving his initial prognosis of six months by about five years. In 1993, Michael Jackson recorded a song—"Gone Too Soon"—to commemorate him.

White's legacy was sealed with the 1990 legislation that bore his name. White never disassociated himself from the numerous gay men who were suffering the same condition as he, and his activism provided a media story that the broader public could empathize with. His compassion for other AIDS victims garnered adoration not only from celebrities like Jackson, Elizabeth Taylor, and Elton John, but also from the LGBTQ community (we always love a good ally). White gave cover for politicians to finally support funding to care for people living with AIDS. Although advocacy from AIDS providers and activists had paved a long and arduous road toward its passage, it was not a coincidence that the CARE Act ultimately commemorated a White teenager from the Midwest who was a hemophiliac, the most "innocent" of the so-called four Hs (the other three being homosexuals, heroin addicts, and Haitians). The support for the CARE Act was so strong in Congress that it was veto proof. (In the Senate, the bill had sixty-six cosponsors and ninety-five senators voted in favor of it.) President George H. W. Bush, a frequent target of ACT UP demonstrations, had no choice but to rescind his initial opposition to the bill and sign it into law in August, 1990, just months after White's death. The CARE Act finally provided major federal funding for AIDS services. Having been reauthorized several times since, the program continues to this day.

The initial AIDS demonstration grants in 1986 went to only four cities. Its equivalent (Title I) under the CARE Act in the first round in 1991 awarded sixteen cities. Total funding in 1991 exceeded $220 million, more than ten times the amount of HRSA's first effort of AIDS funding five years before. But more than funding, the CARE Act also changed the role local grassroots activists played in how these public dollars would be allocated in their respective city. HRSA required each jurisdiction receiving CARE Act funding to create a "planning council" to "identify service needs and gaps, develop plans for HIV delivery, and establish priorities for funding allocations."

The advocacy by AIDS activists of color at GMOCC paid off just in time for the 1990 passage of the Ryan White CARE Act. The legislation required any county receiving a grant to establish an "HIV Health Services Planning Council"—but without specifying "what level of detail the Planning Council will have authority to prioritize," according to meeting minutes by the LA County AIDS Commission. By November,

Robert Gates, director of the LA County Department of Health Services, had outlined options available to the board of supervisors. Gates suggested that the planning council be responsible for "establish[ing] priorities for the allocation of funds within the eligible area" and "assess[ing] the efficiency of the administrative mechanism in rapidly allocating funds to the areas of greatest need in the eligible area." He also proposed that the planning council comprise eighteen members from the existing AIDS commission, six representatives from government agencies, and fourteen at-large members representing different communities affected by the epidemic. As a result, GMOCC agency members had seats on the council, including Dean, representing the Asian American community. Phill, who had become the AIDS coordinator for the city of LA, served as its first cochair, along with Suzi Rodriguez, a Latina AIDS activist. AIDS commissioner Dr. Mark Katz acknowledged that the council makeup was "an important accomplishment in the community, in terms of grassroots activists meeting with people representing administration" on equal footing. Phill attributed this feat to the increasing clout of AIDS activists of color. "Because of the work we [GMOCC] had done, it certainly influenced seats on the council," he said. "When the council was first comprised, it reflected that kind of diversity. The heads of the Los Angeles County HIV Planning Council were a HIV-positive Black gay man and a Latina!" In 1993, the planning council made permanent institutional seats for seven entities. Some were powerhouses, like APLA, GLCSC, and AIDS Healthcare Foundation. But organizations serving underserved populations were also allotted permanent seats, including Altamed and MAP. Institutional seats were also reserved for an agency serving women with HIV and another representing the Asian American community. (To avoid overlap, the AIDS commission and the planning council later combined into one entity called the Los Angeles County Commission on HIV.)

After the makeup of the planning council had been established, the next big decision was funding priorities. The federal legislation specified certain services. Some were obvious, like outpatient medical care, outreach for testing, and mental health/psychosocial services. Others were left to be defined by local needs. Council members had to agree on how much of the federal funding would be allocated to each category. "Everything was contentious back then," said Phill. "Literally everything."

Both he and Oscar recalled the same controversial incident. Phill said, "There was an organization called PAWS, Pets Are Wonderful Support. They came to the council wanting funding for pets to provide emotional support to people living with HIV. The people of color were like, 'Are you freaking kidding us? We can't get people housing or meds or food and you want us to spend money on dog food? Only in West Hollywood would this even come up.'"

In the beginning, the people of color on the council were frustrated that not a lot of money was earmarked for their communities. That didn't mean these activists were concerned the only with the needs of gay men of color. In one instance, Oscar recalled that the GMOCC joined the women on the council in advocating against the elimination of childcare as a funding category. Unfortunately, as Oscar said, "All of these conversations would take place in the same environment where other people were advocating for pets for people living with HIV." Both Phill and Oscar acknowledged that the services provided by PAWS were legitimate, but as cochair, Phill had to balance this request with all the others. Phill said, "I was known for saying to the council, every decision we make to do something is a decision not to do something else."

When the nonprofit AIDS infrastructure was suddenly flooded with millions in new funding, activists had hoped that the CARE Act would usher in a more equitable funding approach. As Larry Harold expressed at an AIDS commission meeting in February, 1991, the funding priorities should consider "underserved" and "hard-hit" areas, with more money going to community-based organizations "rather than to continue to fund public or county-based organizations as has been done in the past." The funding cycle in the first year reflected some success of this advocacy. GMOCC received funding for cross-training for staff as well as outreach and promotion of services. MAP, which had a longer history than their GMOCC peers in providing HIV services, won a contract for mental health and psychosocial support, and the Asian Pacific AIDS Education Project received a modest amount of $25,000 for translation services.

Funding for Bienestar and APAIT was coming in more slowly. Initially, they were relegated to a smaller pool of money for outreach and prevention. Any public health professional would tell you that prevention was absolutely crucial in stemming an epidemic, and as subsequent chapters will show, APAIT staff initiated some innovative social marketing campaigns with the limited resources. But our health-care system has always prioritized treating a disease over preventing it. Providing direct services to people with HIV, such as treatment and counseling, requires staff with advanced degrees and professional credentials, as well as office set-up, information technology, and policies and procedures that safeguard client confidentiality. For organizations like Bienestar and APAIT, it was a chicken-or-egg dilemma. Without this infrastructure, they couldn't be competitive in getting more public funding; without more funding, they couldn't improve their infrastructure.

Oscar said, "They always asked, do you guys have the capacity? Of course, they never questioned our cultural competence because that was clear. They could see that all of us had strong connections [to our communities] and could deliver." In fact, many mainstream organizations depended on these connections as a pipeline to deliver hard-to-reach clients whom they otherwise couldn't find. To them, that was the perfect arrangement, a status quo that would keep competition for direct services dollars minimal and manageable.

But Oscar and Dean had other ideas. They didn't want to stay in their lanes. Because the planning council could create new service categories for funding, they pushed for a category in capacity building. Their argument was that in order to serve these neglected communities fully, the county needed to support building the capacity of those organizations that had deep roots in these communities, like Bienestar and APAIT. "They told us we'd never get money for case management," Ric recalled. "Or for treatment advocacy. They told us that would never happen. The naysayers will crush your dreams if you let them. We did a lot of advocacy. They didn't just hand us the money. We had to go to the HIV commission and say, 'Look, we need these resources for our community, and it's your responsibility to allocate resources that are equitable and fair.' If it hadn't been us making some noise, nobody would pay attention to the API community." GMOCC also worked their public officials, and they found an ally in John Schunhoff, the director of the Office of AIDS in LA, who was committed to serving people of color and women. All these insider-outsider tactics paid off, and the council approved the capacity funding. The growth didn't happen overnight, but the movement finally had the fuel it needed to take off.

CHAPTER 7

The Young and the Fearless

A SIAN PACIFIC AIDS INTERVENTION TEAM (APAIT) HAD MOVED to Special Service for Groups (SSG) just as federal money was starting to stream into LA County. The agency couldn't compete with the big fish yet. APAIT still didn't provide direct services, and it was serving a relatively small target population. Yet their advocacy with other communities of color meant that they were at least getting more money to hire staff beyond the trinity of cofounders, Dean Goishi, Ric Parish, and Joël Tan. The people they found were young (often just coming out of college, if they had graduated at all) and willing to work for the low pay the agency offered. But they were not a desperate bunch. In fact, these young people felt called to do this work. Diep Tran, who joined the staff in the mid-1990s, said, "We didn't really care about stability, longevity. We just wanted to do work that animated us, work that changed culture and moved it forward. We didn't care about [our] survival."

In exchange for this enthusiasm and energy, APAIT offered young activists a space to develop a politicized queer identity. "It allowed people to work out their LGBTQ identity by focusing on something else besides sexuality," Eric Reyes said. "And they could do all this with the help of the resources behind these organizations."

J Craig Fong explained it this way:

There was a generational shift. If you were born in the fifties and before, your goal for gay rights was just, "Please don't beat me up, leave me alone." That would have been good enough. Well, for the generation after that, those born in the mid-sixties, seventies, that's not good enough. [Then came] the election of Bill Clinton [in 1992]. It wasn't necessarily because of Clinton the man himself, but because people felt, after all these years of Reagan and Bush, they could finally poke their noses out of the closet. Clinton came along and said, "You should be allowed to serve in the military." Whether you were gay or lesbian or HIV positive or both, or a person of color, the Clinton administration gave us the feeling that we didn't have to be quite as afraid as much as we were. And in '93, there was the huge March on Washington [for Lesbian, Gay, and Bi Equal Rights]. People were standing together shoulder to shoulder. Suddenly there was this efflorescence, this bursting out. More people were willing to fight.

Sally Jue explained the generational difference similarly: "I don't think they [young people] experienced gay stigma in the same way. They were more willing to be out. Many of them were starting to retake owner-ship of the word *queer*. Their gay coming of age was tied to the HIV epi-demic. That was how they were being political, as opposed to something like Stonewall. There was that greater sense of urgency and a much clearer mission."

Just as Joël and Ric predicted when they were organizing young people in Colors United, AIDS became a central issue for this generation of LGBTQ Asian American activists to rally around.

The first person APAIT hired, after joining SSG, was Unhei Kang, a Korean-American bisexual woman. After Unhei received her bachelor's degree in social work from California State University, Long Beach, she found a job as an AIDS case manager at Project Ahead in the same city. "I worked predominantly with gay men, the homeless population, and per-sons with drug issues," she explained. "My job was primarily helping them with financial issues, like rental or utility assistance, or hooking them up with various services. And listening to them." The men at Project Ahead thought "it was really sweet that a straight young Asian woman was will-ing to do this work." Unhei had to remind them that she was bisexual and had a girlfriend. With a circle of friends who were mostly LGBTQ, Unhei fell into this line of work because she felt a sense of camaraderie with those who were either afflicted or at high risk for AIDS. She said, "Being a bi woman, being ostracized by my family for my sexuality, helped me to empathize and want to provide support and to educate."

Around that time, Unhei remembered meeting Ric and Joël at a local conference for Asian American community-based organizations. They were on the same panel presenting on LGBTQ issues. Afterward, they asked her if she'd be interested in volunteering for APAIT. She replied, "Sure. Why not?" Soon she "was hanging out a lot in front of gay clubs, passing out condoms and pamphlets and trying to educate the community that everyone is at risk for HIV/AIDS." Unhei also remembered doing outreach at "underground parties in industrial neighborhoods." "Once Ric also took me to a bath house [for outreach]," she added, laughing. She wasn't the only woman who volunteered with APAIT. Unhei recalled other women—straight, lesbian, and bi—"who wanted to help our brothers." Not all her outreach targeted gay men, either. The outreach sometimes took Unhei to straight clubs, where she would find young Asian American women confiding in her about pregnancy or STD concerns. This experience made Unhei "realize that there's a need for not just HIV/AIDS education [for women], but also education about STD and birth control." On the ground, she saw the same intersection between AIDS and reproductive health that Lisa Hasegawa saw (discussed in chapter 5), an intersection that funding silos often obscured. In the agency, she was among the first to advocate more resources to promote women's sexual health in a field that was dominated by gay male voices.

A year later, Unhei quit her job in Long Beach to start a master's program in social work at UCLA. But since she was putting herself through school, she still needed to work. When APAIT offered her a part-time job, she took it. Initially, her job description included grant writing, fundraising, and volunteer recruitment. And because the agency was still so small—all hands were always on deck—she continued to take part in community outreach. Her negative experience with her family drove her commitment to the work. "I felt very protective of the clients, of the people that were coming through [APAIT]," she said. "Even though I was young, I felt like a mother hen. It was upsetting for me that people were getting ostracized from their family. I just didn't think it was fair."

APAIT soon received some funding for a woman's program, which Unhei ran initially. Around the same time, she and a group of Asian

American lesbians and bisexual women cofounded Los Angeles Asian Pacific Islander Sisters (LAAPIS). As discussed in a later chapter, her activism through APAIT and LAAPIS would merge, becoming yet another example of how AIDS activism fueled community building for the broader LGBTQ Asian American population in LA.

Noel Alumit was barely a teenager when he heard of AIDS in the early 1980s. Even at that young age, he was certain that he was gay, and the news of the disease "intrigued" him. AIDS informed the way he moved through this world for many years to come, even without being HIV positive. "I knew that it was lurking out there," he explained, "and to some degree it affirmed there was maybe something wrong with being LGBT, that there was this disease that was coming after us. . . . There was this impending doom or badness that was coming. It colored the way I saw the world and maybe even how the world saw me."

As he became older, Noel was weighed down by this "incredible amount of unfairness" so much that he started "dabbling" in sex and alcohol as a way to avoid his "grief." Now he could recognize the irony of sexual ecstasy as a way to feel numb. But for a generation of young men who were coming out in the age of AIDS, the script was all too familiar. As a theater major at the University of Southern California, he began to learn another script. Noel auditioned for a student production of *As Is*, by William Hoffman, one of the first Broadway plays about AIDS. He was going for one of the lead characters that was originally written as White and Jewish. Noel recalled, "I did a great job in the audition, but they wanted me to take a lesser role because both the lead characters in the play were White." Arguing that the sexuality of the characters was "something [he] authentically connected to," Noel fought for the role that he eventually got. "This wasn't just another play," he said. "No, this was a gay character in an AIDS play. The other actors who did audition for it were not gay. That was a turning point for me. Chances are, back then, this might be the only gay character I would ever play."

That wouldn't be the last time Noel played a gay character in an AIDS play; he was also featured in Chay Yew's *A Language of Their Own* in the play's 1994 premiere in LA. But he considered his role in *As Is* at USC his first AIDS work in what would turn out to be a remarkably long career in this field (for a while, Noel was the longest-serving employee at APAIT, at almost two decades). For "research," the cast took a field trip to West Hollywood for a dose of gay life. But it was during rehearsals where Noel began to develop his empathy toward those living with the virus. He said, "We took weeks to develop our characters. We did a lot of processing in the development of this play: delving into these characters and how they feel and what it's like to have a partner who's HIV positive, what it's like to live in a world where people may not like you, so to be able to experience that as a creative person. It did provide me with a kind of compassion to do AIDS work later on, because I wasn't as afraid."

Shortly after the play, newly sober as the 1980s rolled into the 1990s, Noel became more involved in the recovery community. There, he met people who were living with the virus, as there was a high correlation between drug use and HIV infection. After he graduated, as he was searching for work as an actor, Noel volunteered for the Chris Brownlie Hospice, the first AIDS hospice in California that was opened by what is now called the AIDS Healthcare Foundation. (Brownlie was Phill Wilson's longtime partner, who passed away from AIDS complications shortly after the hospice in his namesake was opened the day after Christmas in 1988. The twenty-five-bed hospice would stay in operation until 1996.) His sister, also a volunteer at the hospice, recruited Noel. For an out-of-work recent graduate, a sudden overabundance of unstructured time was "not a good thing if you're newly sober," Noel said. "I needed something to keep me busy, to give me a set schedule. Volunteer work was that."

The hospice was "eye-opening." Until then, Noel had been fed by the media that AIDS was a gay White man's disease. Noel recalled:

When I walked into this hospice, there were all these people of color and women. There was a Filipina who looked like one of the aunts I grew up with. That was like, wow. I had no idea. No idea. I was compartmentalizing my life. "This is my gay life, and that is my Filipino life." In that moment seeing her, it all came together. Where is the Filipino family that should be here? I thought people of color had these extended families. Black, Latino, Asian, we have big gatherings. We have cousins for miles. I thought to myself, "But people are dying alone. What is wrong here?" To see that Filipina woman there, who on the street you would never, ever know, had AIDS. . . . And she was in the last six months of her life . . .

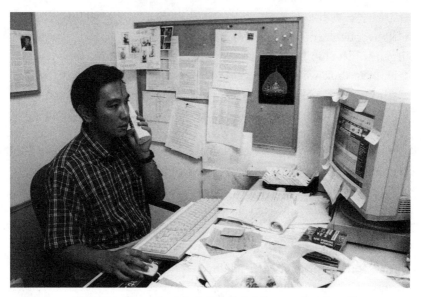

FIGURE 7.1. APAIT staff member Noel Alumit fielding a call at the office. Courtesy of APAIT, a division of Special Service for Groups, Inc.

At a loss for words, Noel eventually summarized, "'eye-opening' is an understatement."

The hospice experience added a new dimension of his racial and ethnic identity to his fledgling AIDS work. To bring together his creative side with his activist one, Noel found a part-time job at the LA Free Clinic, which was experimenting with AIDS education through theater, in what they called Project ABLE, AIDS Beliefs Learned through Education. The troupe would book gigs at "youth-populated places"—anywhere from high schools to halfway houses with abused children and to the California Youth Authority correctional facilities and camps—and performed a series of AIDS education sketches. Noel remembered playing in front of a group of teen moms. They chose a play about how a pregnant woman with HIV could minimize the risk of passing on the virus to her fetus. After the performance, everyone in the audience got tested for HIV. Noel also found work at East West Player, the premier Asian American theater in LA.

In 1993, he joined APAIT (figure 7.1). At the interview, Dean Goishi and Naomi Kageyama asked him, "Are you comfortable going to bars and bathhouses and sex clubs and bushes?" (The last referred to public sex environments, like parks, where many men who have sex with men could find each other anonymously.)

He thought to himself, "You're going to pay me to do this?" His actual reply? "I was there last weekend!"

Like many young gay men grappling with their sexuality in the early 1980s, Napoleon Lustre first learned about AIDS in the form of a terrible joke. "What do you call a faggot on roller skates?" asked Napoleon's coworker at Burger King in 1982, where the sixteen-year-old had just landed a part-time job. "Rolaids." It wasn't the first time Napoleon had heard someone put down gay people, but he wasn't identifying as gay at that point, even though he knew he was attracted to men. Identity was never straightforward for Napoleon. He was always adjacent to something else. Born in the Philippines in 1965, he immigrated to the US at the age of twelve. Ask him what his ethnicity is, and he'll tell you "I'm Filipino with an F. I'm Asian, but I'm not. I'm Pacific Islander, but I'm not. I'm Latino, but I'm not. That's always what I feel about being Filipino." Gayness was not something he was gravitating toward as a teenager. "I was tormented about my sexuality," Napoleon said of those formative years. "I had shut down sexually. I wasn't making out with anybody, boy or girl." So he didn't take that AIDS joke very seriously.

At the time, Napoleon was living with his older sister in Bellflower. The two would hang out and go clubbing at a sixteen-and-over dance club called Infinity in Long Beach. "There was a bar called Forced Heat close by," he recalled vividly. "It was a leather bar. I remember just gawking in there secretly and seeing these men in black leather. It was smoky and it smelled raunchy. It just excited me." His uncle had also taken Napoleon to Pickwick Bookshop on Hollywood Boulevard when he was younger, where he found "paperbacks of gay novels that were popular at the time." Young Napoleon thought, "If there were gay books there, there were gay people around." He stored all this information in his head until he could explore the city on his own.

That time came soon enough when as a high school senior, he learned how to drive. "I would borrow my sister's car and drive to the parts of town that I knew gay men hung out in West Hollywood," he reported. "I would hang out in Vaseline Alley, outside, behind the Gold Coast Bar, with a lot of punks and runaways and prostitutes. That was my hangout until four or five in the morning. I would try to go into the bars, and sometimes they would kick me out." When he was successful in wrangling his way into a bar, he "would buy a beer and nurse it all night."

All this furtive lurking finally led to his first sexual encounter. By this time, Napoleon was a student at University of California, Irvine (UCI). Even though his life had moved further into Orange County, he was still making his trek to West Hollywood. One night, in Vaseline Alley, Napoleon was cruising another man until the man went into the Gold Coast. At the end of the night, he came stumbling out drunk. Napoleon said, "We finally talked and he took me home. He lived just around the corner. That's where I had my first full-on gay sex."

It turned out to be much more than a one-night stand. Napoleon became involved with this man for a year and a half. His lover had served during the Vietnam War, but, at a base in Japan, never saw any fighting. What he got out of the war, though, was information about the burgeoning gay community back home. "After he came home in the seventies," Napoleon said, "he blossomed with the gay subculture." The man was thirty-four, almost twice the age of Napoleon. "I always preferred older men. I always used to say, 'Older men have better stories.' I couldn't be bothered with young guys."

The relationship distracted Napoleon's academic career. Having come into UCI as a "promising A student," he almost had to drop out. In his freshman year, Napoleon remembered succinctly, he received two Cs, two Ds, and two Fs. "I tried, but I was going to West Hollywood and spending time with him," he explained, "because that was the first time that I had a space where I was out, I was among gay culture. It was very utopian. College was utopian, too, but they were competing utopias." He did try to reconcile the two by "working out his queer identity" on campus. He joined the Gay and Lesbian Student Union at UCI and even took a leadership position as the cochair after a couple of years. There was a large and organized Filipino student population at the university as well, but he hadn't felt close to them. "They were a bunch of straight eggheads," he said. "They had a Filipino culture night at the big auditorium [on campus] and they did an anti-gay joke. It fucking pissed me off. I walked out. They expected me to be active with them, and they did shit like that?"

Off campus, his relationship came to an end when his lover's life fell apart. All the signs were pointing to him being an alcoholic, but

Napoleon was too young to notice them. "I thought he just made a drink at 10 a.m. because that was what people do. I was sheltered and naïve in a way." The man moved back to his family in Arkansas.

In his third year at UCI (and still a freshman by units), Napoleon was heeding a local public health campaign to get tested for HIV. Napoleon and his roommate decided to go together. He said, "We went to the public health clinic in Santa Ana. Two weeks later, he said to me, 'I got my results. I'm negative.' And I said nothing, because I hadn't gotten my result yet." Finally, with an older man he was dating at the time, he gathered up the courage to go back to the clinic.

The result came back positive. Napoleon was barely twenty-one.

"It was a shock," he said repeatedly.

There's always a possibility, but it was a shock. The guy I was dating was really cool about it. He left me alone in my silence on the drive home. I got really depressed, I froze. I told one person who was my best friend from high school. Big White girl. Being the fag I was, I was best friends with the big girl. She told somebody, and it spread like wildfire. There was a network of people that knew about me, and I wasn't aware [they knew]. It still pisses me off. At least they were good people who didn't use it against me, to hurt me somehow. I was lucky, but it was such dangerous information. You got to really guard it.

The news about his HIV status came at a time when his queer identity was becoming more emboldened. He participated in the Second National March on Washington for Gay and Lesbian Rights in 1987. His best friend bought him a plane ticket as his birthday present that October. He said, "We overran the city. We took the subway to the march, and everybody was queer. ACT UP was there. Whoopi Goldberg was marching with PWA [people with AIDS]. The next day we went to the Supreme Court to protest the [Bowers v.] Hardwick decision [where the Supreme Court upheld a Georgia sodomy law outlawing anal and oral sex between consenting adults]." At the march, he witnessed DC police wearing yellow gloves in anticipation of interacting with people with HIV. The crowd chanted back, "Your gloves don't match your shoes!" "It was so funny," said Napoleon. "The humor of the activists was so refreshing, and I thought, 'This is my fucking revolution.' I loved it so much because it just fired me up. They told me I was gonna die in three years average. I was like, 'Fuck it. Let's make this life significant.' I wanted to fight."

Coming back from the nation's capital, Napoleon successfully ran for the cochair position at the Gay and Lesbian Student Union. That post gave him an opportunity to learn community organizing. He worked closely with the Graduate Student Association, which was led by a progressive gay man, to lobby the university to extend its on-campus family housing to queer couples. He was part of a delegation that met with the chancellor and fought all the way to the board of regents of the entire University of California system. Through his tenure, they won some demands, like a resource center for LGBTQ students, but they weren't able to change the housing policy. The loss was "heartbreaking," but the struggle invigorated Napoleon at a time when he didn't expect to live more than a couple of years.

"No one has more energy than the dying," he said. "Young people are already fearless, right? I was fearless in my youth, but I was also dying. So I was doubly fearless. You can't threaten a young person who's dying."

He was getting sick once in a while, enough to make him fall behind in his school work. But he wasn't dying. His activist work enlivened him. It was definitely more exciting and meaningful than any papers he had to write for a diploma. Eventually, he dropped out of college.

The road to wellness had a few missteps. Early on in his diagnosis, he sought out a support group for people with HIV in Orange County. "I walked into the wrong room, and I ended up in the room of the support group for caregivers for people with AIDS. One guy shared how he was dreading Christmas and how he wanted his love to die because he couldn't deal with another Christmas again. That was the first thing I heard. I was appreciating their honesty, of course, but that was not the room for me. That was something else." Even when he found the right group, he found himself sitting in a room with forty- or fifty-year-old White men. The conversation was "isolating" to him, even though these groups were all he had.

By the early 1990s, five years living with HIV, he was even dating. Not an older man this time, but a younger Vietnamese American. One day, the two were in a bakery in West Hollywood when an Asian man approached them and started a conversation. It was Joël Tan.

Napoleon quickly saw what people already knew about the APAIT cofounder. "Joël is a community builder. He finds communities. He builds communities," he said. Joël recruited him to be a volunteer at APAIT. Game recognizing game, Joël saw how good Napoleon would be at outreach. And the agency needed more staff who were HIV positive if they wanted to get more serious about working with people who were directly affected by the virus beyond outreach and education. A volunteer gig turned into a paying one. Along with Noel, Napoleon was one of the earliest community health outreach workers at APAIT.

In addition to the more mainstream gay bars and disco clubs, Napoleon would also hit the seedier bathhouses and sex clubs, looking primarily for Filipino gay men in these spaces. The nonjudgmental approach in general HIV outreach was even more important for these patrons. Napoleon knew how "to normalize whatever is happening so that people feel completely at ease with their own decisions as they're making them." But that wasn't enough. The usual method just wasn't working for him. "It was dead, from the get-go," Napoleon said.

> You couldn't just have a table and wait for them to come to you. The "good boys" would come to you. They wanted condoms. The ones that didn't were those that were going to stay away from you because they didn't want to have that conversation. You're filtering against your own objectives just by the location. I would go into the bathhouse, talk to people in the rooms. I would go in and have a conversation. You make relationships. You don't expect a connection until four or five encounters later. But you develop it because it's a really important relationship.

Posing as a patron to infiltrate the establishment was not protocol, but Napoleon had a strong opinion about that. "The protocol was bullshit. The protocol was idiotic. They were written by bureaucrats who had no field experience. At the same time, nobody knew what they were doing, so it didn't really matter. Everybody was a novice. We fucked up a lot and we corrected each other's mistakes, and we fought with each other over stuff. It was all just part of the war."

Born in Maui, Hawai'i, Tracy Nako moved to LA in late 1987, when he was in his mid-twenties. Tracy had a taste of gay life in Waikiki, but like his social network at the time, which was made up entirely of people who were gay and from Hawai'i, Tracy had come to the mainland to "escape" his home state. "It was a little bit repressive," he explained, "being in Hawai'i, being closeted and fearing that if someone saw you walking into a gay bar, that you would be rejected by your family. For a lot of us, moving to the mainland was liberating." At first, he was living in Torrance and working at an advertising agency in the San Fernando Valley, many miles and a few freeways to the north. The long commute didn't deter him from experiencing gay life in the bigger city. He recalled, "The first couple years in Los Angeles was like, Wow! All these gay bars and we partied three or four times a week." Each time, he and his friends hit a different spot. "Usually we went with a group and we also went home as a group. I wasn't having a lot of sex. It was more about partying and being young and gay in a big city." Even though the epidemic was on its way to its summit in the late 1980s, Tracy admitted he "wasn't that attuned to the risk." One of his good friends, who Tracy found out later was HIV positive, joined ACT UP, and Tracy went to different demonstrations with him. At that time, AIDS was more of a "political thing."

By 1991, Tracy wanted to do "less partying." He started volunteering with the AIDS Project Los Angeles (APLA), the most notable of AIDS service organizations, as a buddy to an African American man living with HIV in South LA. He also made a career change and started working for the Asian American Drug Abuse Program (AADAP). AADAP was (and still is) headquartered in South LA. South LA was the epicenter of the CIA-fueled crack epidemic, which by the time Tracy joined the organization was at its tail end (though the impact would be felt for many years following). As a result, AADAP had a substantial client population of African Americans who were at risk of HIV. Tracy was hired as a substance abuse counselor, and he made it part of his job to bring HIV education to AADAP's client population. The agency was receptive, and Tracy found support among other younger and more open-minded staff for his initiative.

In his HIV work, he met Dean Goishi, when the AIT was still part of Asian Pacific Lesbians and Gays (A/PLG). Dean invited Tracy to an A/PLG function, and Tracy eventually switched from volunteering with APLA to AIT. In 1993, Tracy was hired as a case manager at APAIT, when the agency finally received county funding to work directly with the HIV-positive population. Tracy remembered "starting off very small and very slow." There were fewer than twenty clients in the first year, but the case management services were intense. Tracy said, "I would go to people's homes to protect their privacy. And people lived all over the county!" He went out of his way to provide a vital service to limited English proficient clients who otherwise would highly likely drop a treatment program in a mainstream organization. Now having a track record of working with the HIV-positive population, with a niche in cultural and linguistic responsiveness in the Asian immigrant communities, APAIT would go on to broaden its portfolio of direct services, first to include treatment advocacy, and then mental health counseling.

Regardless of their job titles, these young staff members pounded the pavement all over LA after hours for outreach. Along the way, they recruited an army of volunteers, many of them, like myself, drafted from queer student organizations from local college campuses. APAIT's community outreach took us to diverse spaces in different communities, but the focus was on venues where gay Asian men congregated. Since the late 1970s, there had been a handful of establishments that catered mostly to gay Asian men (and their admirers). As larger-scale dance clubs began to clutter the streets of West Hollywood, a new generation of gay Asian men began to flood "Boys Town," to the point where some mainstream bars started to have an "Asian night" on a regular basis. Later in the 1990s, promoters organized gay Asian parties in non-traditional venues, like Red Dragon at the El Rey Theater, that would draw hundreds of gay Asian men every month.

APAIT staff set up tables outside, with educational materials and safer-sex packets to greet patrons entering and leaving these venues. After some training and an orientation, we volunteers took our clipboards and approached anyone who looked Asian with a "quick survey." We asked them a few questions about HIV; for instance, what are the four ways HIV could be transmitted? (Blood, semen, breast milk, and pre-cum.) We supplied the right answers when they couldn't come up with them and corrected misconceptions. That was the kind of encounter APAIT could count toward their goal for their public contracts. The whole process could be very transactional. So our ears perked up if they asked us a question—the possibility of a conversation, a deeper connection.

Some people, like Noel, a self-described "chatterbox," were very good at opening up a dialogue with the club goers. And in a town where gay Asian men were rendered invisible, Noel met many of them "who were starving for friends." But just because it was becoming easier to find gay Asian men, it didn't mean the gay Asian men would skip and bounce and fall over themselves to talk to the APAIT staff and volunteers about using condoms and the possibility of catching HIV, in environments where drinking and hooking up was the happy purpose of the evening. Sometimes the bar owners were the ones who resisted the most. Ric remembered doing outreach at Mugi's, a dive bar that used to cater to gay Asian men on Hollywood Boulevard, in the heart of what is now Thai Town. He said, "The [Japanese] owner flat out told us, 'I don't want you scaring our customers with all this AIDS stuff.' Somehow we got him to give us a quiet little corner [laughs] . . . to hand out condoms and information, but they didn't like it at all." Other times, the problematic dynamics between White and Asian gay men got in the way of an outreach encounter. Ric recalled, "We were talking to this one kid. He looked like he was about twenty. He was looking at our pamphlets. He was interested. All of a sudden, his White lover came and snatched [the pamphlet] out of his hand and handed it back to us. He said, 'He doesn't need that.' And he pulled him away. In that moment, that's when we realized what we were up against."

I had a similar encounter when the White lover of an Asian man I was talking to interrupted our conversation. But instead of being mean, he actually started talking to me casually. It took the confused me a while before I realized he was flirting with me, in front of his boyfriend. These incidents happened often enough that the staff covered these scenarios in the volunteers' orientation.

Even without any obstacles, many people needed more than one approach to feel comfortable trusting a stranger with their questions about the most intimate part of their lives. APAIT volunteers and staff stationed at these venues regularly until they became a constant presence. Sometimes it helped to switch up the outreach team. Unhei thought that a female volunteer or staff member would be less threatening to some gay Asian men. Surprisingly, staff also took advantage of this White-Asian dynamic that they were trying to push back. Eric Reyes remembered a White volunteer named Chuck who was particularly effective in talking to Asian men.

"He was our token White guy," said Eric. "And he totally understood the racial politics. But he didn't take advantage of it [for his personal gains]. He understood that Asian gay men at that time would respond to a White male coming to talk with them more than to another gay Asian man. If it was just three Asian men at a table, it'd be pretty tough for them to approach. [Chuck] was more than willing to be our White guy."

Joël appreciated the contradictions in leveraging a Whiteness that reaffirmed the racial hierarchy in the community. "We wanted to be future facing, but we had to meet people where they were at," he said. Despite being one of the loudest critics of A/PLG, he advocated White volunteers doing outreach to Asian men. "We couldn't moralize anybody into healthy behavior."

The goal of one-on-one prevention outreach was twofold. First, because unprotected sex was the likeliest transmission route for men who have sex with men, the outreach focused on convincing this high-risk population to use a condom, especially for anal sex. Joël knew in the eighties the case for condoms was hard to make to a population for whom free and intimate exchange of fluids between men was almost a requisite definition of gayness. "That's one way of understanding 'natural,' at least in my generation," he said. And a condom was anything but that. But as Napoleon added, "The condom was king. That's all we had at that time. There were some controversies about how contagious pre-cum was, whether oral sex was medium or low risk. Part of the education was to really let people understand and feel out how connected they wanted to be and how to negotiate those risks. Like you decide, are you going to suck a dick without condom? People had to make these really personal decisions." In those days, the hope for a cure was almost just as infectious as the virus itself. "Some of us urged men [to use condoms] by saying it's fun and different and it's only for the duration," Joël remembered. "When they find the cure, we can go back to being normal." But the light of an AIDS cure faded with each year as the mortality rate rose and clinical trials turned their attention to medications that tried to manage the symptoms rather than eliminate the cause. Condoms, for my generation that came of age in the early 1990s, had become the new normal.

Second, outreach encouraged these men to get tested. If someone was positive, knowing their status could influence them to make more responsible decisions when engaging in sex with another person. Early detection could also help these individuals stave off sickness and death. Even if someone tested negative, the act of testing, especially regular testing, could prompt people to think more actively about their health and make healthy decisions to stay negative.

The testing message wasn't more welcomed than the condom one. AIDS had been such a constant throughout the 1980s in the gay community that many people had simply resigned to the almost certain fact that they would contract the virus. Some fatalistic ones preferred denial, and others refused to let the scepter of HIV hang over them at all. In either case, why would they subject themselves to the humiliation and anxieties of HIV testing? At that time, there was a one-week lapse between the test and the result. Those feelings of guilt, regrets, and anxieties could linger every waking minute of that week, and many people simply did not return for the result.

So the AIDS activists in the Asian American community not only had to figure out how to get their target population to talk to them, but once these men came to their table, they also had to be creative and innovative in their messaging. Joël acknowledged that "none of us had any background in communication or public health. But we were figuring out what we could convey to our community to get them to be safe during this duration?" It was a time before evidence-based practice became a cottage industry in public health, where a strategy that had proven scientifically to work in one population was replicated, sometimes uncritically, in another. But what these activists lacked in public health experience, they more than made up with their collective understanding of the cultural contexts in the lives of gay Asian men.

Under Joël, the team came up with a couple of ideas of packaging their safer-sex message that juxtaposed familiar cultural symbols in unexpected settings. As a volunteer, I remember stuffing a condom and a tiny tube of lubricant into a red envelope, the kind that is given out during Lunar New Year. Even though the custom was strictly Chinese, it had enough pan-ethnic resonance that even the most closeted gay Asian man coming out of a bar would recognize it and find it hard to resist picking it up. Heng Lam Foong and Connie Wong, an Asian lesbian couple that had separate trajectories with AIDS activism in LA, both remembered the red envelope safer-sex packets vividly. Heng said, "[Red envelopes are] very auspicious. You're using something that has a very positive connotation to do outreach, to let people know that you can take care of yourself. I thought it was very clever that it was used to show that it's not all negativity."

Connie recalled a specific outreach event at the Sunset Junction Street Fair, which between 1980 and 2010 (especially in the early years) attracted a diverse crowd of LGBTQ people and immigrants in the pre-gentrified Silverlake neighborhood (imagine leather daddies in chaps walking next to *abuelitas* pushing strollers). Staffing the APAIT booth at the event, Connie saw "two Chinese grandmothers grabbing the red envelopes because they wanted freebies and giggling about it." They had come to the booth specifically for that. If it was safe enough for the grandmothers, men who were not open about their sexuality shouldn't feel intimidated about picking it up.

Another example is putting messages about where to get tested in fortune cookies. Though a stateside invention, most Asian immigrants recognized what it was. Refusing a fortune cookie was almost like turning away good luck. Napoleon credited Joël and Ric with this kind of innovation. He said, "Between the two of them, it was one brilliant idea after another. It was always like a fire catching."

"It was very groundbreaking," said Lisa Hasegawa, who had accompanied Joël to buy the red envelopes in Chinatown. In another time, done by a different group of people, the grab-bag of ethnic artifacts might be construed as cultural appropriation. Joël now called it "anthropological massacre." Lisa recalled that "Joël was like, 'I don't care if they think the red envelopes were sacred. We're doing it.' That was controversial to some people, but people picked it up. That was the point exactly. You just had to push the envelope in those days. I learned to be bold and creative from Joël."

Lisa went to graduate school in public health not too long after this. When she started learning about social marketing, or the use of commercial marketing techniques to encourage people to adopt healthy behavior or improve their environments, she immediately recognized that this was what the APAIT staff had been doing all along.

Red envelopes and fortune cookies were tame compared to what these self-starters did with their media campaigns.

CHAPTER 8

Filthy, Dirty Ads

THE AIDS EPIDEMIC DEVASTATED THE CREATIVE COMMUNITY from the beginning. Sarah Schulman, cofounder of Lesbian Avengers and a member of ACT UP/NY, argued in her book *Gentrification of the Mind* that the death of so many LGBTQ artists in Greenwich Village turned many rent-controlled units vacant and gave way to the gentrification of that neighborhood. The creative community was so irreversibly decimated that it had a ripple effect on the next generation of aspiring artists. Noel Alumit, a budding actor and writer in the early 1990s, said that "there were supposed to be gay artists who would help younger artists become better. Unfortunately, the gay artists who could've done that were dying. Or their lovers or friends were sick, so they could not be there as much as they could have been. My generation of artists who were coming up missed some really great opportunities to work with incredible people." Noel acknowledged many lesbian artists and writers—Ayofemi Falayon, for one—who filled that mentorship role for him. Yet he continued to ponder the break between generations of gay male artists that AIDS had brought on. "A lot of us artists were struggling in the dark," he recalled. "This is not to say my generation of artists were not mature or talented or skilled. We certainly are that. But I do wonder what it may have looked like if there were more men there to shepherd us through."

The Asian American community lost to AIDS a handful of gay artists who had been instrumental to the burgeoning arts and cultural movement that countered mainstream media that continued to perpetrate negative stereotypes about Asians. In 1978, artist Nobuko Miyamoto founded Great Leap to showcase Asian American artists and performers. When Nobuko found out I was working on this book, she wanted to tell me about her good friend, the late actor and choreographer José de Vega, who died of AIDS in 1990. "If I am the mother of Great Leap," Nobuko once said, "José is definitely the father."

Nobuko met José on the set of *West Side Story*. José had played the character Chino in the Academy Award–winning 1961 film, reprising his role in the 1957 Broadway production. Chino was the Shark who was in unrequited love with Maria (his best friend's sister) and later shot and killed Tony, the Romeo to Maria's Juliet in the musical. It was a significant role for the aspiring Filipino American actor and dancer. Under the stage name Joanne Miya, Nobuko played one of Maria's girlfriends. The two would go on to different career paths. José found some success in Hollywood, appearing in a handful of films and gaining worldwide recognition for his choreography. Nobuko, feeling restricted by the mainstream entertainment industry and inspired by the Black Power movement in the 1960s, began to find her own voice and commit to performances that were rooted in her racial and political identities. It was a journey that took her to the founding of Great Leap. In the early 1980s, shortly after that organization was formed, Nobuko and José reconnected at a reunion party for *West Side Story*. She quickly pulled José into her work. José became the principal choreographer and sometimes the director of Great Leap productions (figure 8.1). Nobuko and he composed music and lyrics for the organization's centerpieces, including "Journey in Three Movements" in 1985–86 and "Talk Story I & II" in 1988–89.

In 1986, José found out he was HIV positive and was in and out of the Veterans Hospital. Nobuko visited José every day and witnessed how some staff members were afraid to touch him, and others kept their distance. Despite these restrictions, José continued to work on Great Leap productions up until the last year of his life. Nobuko thought his art was what kept him going. "We were hoping against hope that a cure would happen," she said.

José's indelible influence on the organization continued even after his death. In 1990, partly through the first-voice storytelling movement, Great Leap began to move from group work to showcasing individual artists, such as Jude Narita, Dan Kwong, and Amy Hill, through its

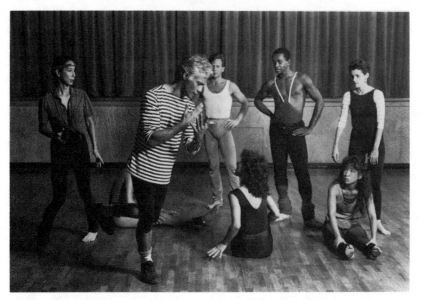

FIGURE 8.1. José de Vega, working on choreography with *Great Leap* cast, including Nobuko Miyamoto (left). Courtesy of Great Leap Archives.

annual production, *A Slice of Rice*. In 1992, in response to the LA Uprising, Great Leap became a "multicultural arts organization which uses art as both performance and creative practice to deepen relations among people of diverse cultures and faiths." Expanding to feature artists from other communities of color, *A Slice of Rice* became *A Slice of Rice, Frijoles and Greens*. Through these evolutions, Nobuko said, "we were trying to be what [José] wanted to be. We were the extension of his mind and creativity."

José wasn't the only artist affiliated with Great Leap to have died of AIDS during that era. Nobuko also remembered Long Nguyen, a dancer in the original slate of *A Slice of Rice* in 1990. Because of his illness, Long cut himself off from the rest of the world in the last two years of his life and lost touch with his artistic community, including Nobuko. In a letter he wrote to her just before he passed away in 1995, he related the process of going from worshiping his healthy dancer's body to hating it, as diarrhea, fatigue, and other complications began to distort it. In the two years that he fell out of touch with Nobuko, he had tried to kill himself. Long wrote, "I was in my complete paranoia world; it was the time for my mind to perform its darkest of dark dances. Incredible!" But as "the wheel of karma turned another notch," he had to learn to love the body and take care of it. He was living in a household of gay men in Amherst, Massachusetts, being cared for primarily by his ex-lover, whom he described as "a bodhisattva who brought me back from the very edge of life." The care slowed the decimation of his body, but the end was unstoppable. Still, Long spoke of a deeper transformation in his final letter to Nobuko: "If I had died then [by killing himself], I wouldn't have been complete. I wouldn't have experienced human love and compassion. I would've died a lonely, incomplete man." He continued, "I believe AIDS was the force that turned the wheel of karma for me. I was knocked out of my selfish, loveless world and lucky enough to have passed through to the next cycle of life. The forces are in balance now."

AIDS took many artists like José and Long from our community, but it also attracted many to the resistance. The influx of AIDS funding in the early 1990s created jobs, especially in community outreach and education, in communities that traditional public health professionals had no inroads into. Artists, seeing the devastation more up close than anyone else, answered the call. The professionalization of the AIDS industry would change this orientation a few years later. In response, some artists became certified as substance abuse counselors or went back to school to become social workers and public health professionals to stay relevant in a field that started to require more credentials. But in the beginning, artists didn't just bring their convictions to the movement, but also their creativity. The gut-wrenching, confrontational, in-your-face messages from the protest movement set the tone for public health messages for HIV prevention in the early 1990s, an innovation for the tamer public health field at the time.

Early on, Asian Pacific AIDS Intervention Team (APAIT) recruited many artists and writers to its staff. Cofounder Joël Tan himself was a writer and performance artist. He organized writing circles, public readings, and slumber parties, where aspiring gay Asian writers like myself could share our work. These events often led to exchanges about navigating the different worlds as proud queer Asians even when these worlds didn't accept all of who we were. Joël considered this community work a significant part of HIV prevention by offering more positive and affirming places for young gay Asian men to go, without resorting to a lot of destructive behavior promoted in mainstream commercial gay spaces.

Other staff also began to experiment with using arts and culture to go beyond the one-on-one outreach model. Noel curated his first "magnet event" at the Abbey, a quiet coffeehouse in West Hollywood that would later be transformed into a bar as the city became more developed. "It was a much smaller Abbey, not the Abbey we know today," Noel said. "I invited performance artist Denise Uyehara and Joël to read, and a Hawaiian dancer [to perform]." Noel carved out time at the event to talk about HIV and the services that APAIT provided. "But the performances were HIV related," he added. "Joël read a poem about AIDS. Denise did something on identity, what it meant to be queer and Asian. And the Hawaiian dancer did a movement on what it was like to experience stigma." APAIT staff also showcased the artwork of Keith Kasai, an outspoken client, at the Abbey. Later on, when Irene Suico Soriano, curator of the Wrestling Tigers reading series, joined the APAIT staff, she would continue this tradition of using literary readings in diverse venues to promote Asian American writers and educate the public about HIV/AIDS and other taboo topics in our community.

As Joël said, "The early movement is an artist-founded movement." Nowhere was this collective creativity more apparent in APAIT than its social marketing campaigns.

Social marketing is similar to commercial marketing. Instead of targeting consumers and asking them to choose one brand over another, social marketing aims to influence a person's behavior to avoid illnesses (prevention) or to seek help if they are already ill (intervention). With stigmatized diseases, social marketing tries to increase community awareness so that people feel more comfortable coming forward for help. The early social marketing campaigns at APAIT were essentially DIY and relied on both the creativity and resourcefulness of staff. There was no money for focus groups to test messages. It helped then that the agency had recruited young and queer Asians who had the pulse of the community, who were themselves not that different from the people they were trying to reach.

The first campaign was rolled out in 1992, just after APAIT had found a home at Special Service for Groups. With some money saved and a small amount Dean was able to get at the discretion of the county Office of AIDS Programs and Policy, Ric was tasked to put together a testing campaign. One night in December 1991, when Ric was hanging out with his friends at a coffeehouse in West Hollywood after an outreach event, they overheard a young Filipino gay man complain, "I wish my nose wasn't so flat. . . . Maybe if I got a nose job, I could score better in West Hollywood." Before Ric could react, he heard someone at his table snap his fingers and retort, "Sistah, love yo Asian body!" Who else could it be but his best friend and comrade, Joël Tan? Ric quickly realized the power of Joël's rejoinder; "Love yo Asian body" encapsulated the lack of sexual agency he saw in the White-Asian dynamics at A/PLG or in front of the bars when they did outreach and explained why it was so hard to talk to other gay Asian men about protecting themselves. "Love Your Asian Body" became APAIT's first social marketing slogan.

In those pre-internet days, the message was propagated through post-cards in one-on-one outreach and advertisements in mass media. There was just enough money in the budget to place ads in the "gay rags," such as *Frontiers, Edge,* and *LN* (Lesbian News), free weeklies that were easily accessible at clubs, bookstores, and coffeehouses that catered to the LGBTQ community. Besides the tagline, "Love Your Asian Body," the postcards and the ads exhorted their audience to get tested for HIV. It was the visual images that captured people's attention and, for some of us, our imagination.

The campaign featured a variety of images of young gay Asian men, in various stages of undress, touching, straddling, embracing, and gazing into one another's eyes (figure 8.2). Ric said of the concept, "It was the first images that we saw of Asian gay men together, making love. Before that, there was always a White guy involved. It was new, and it got a lot of attention." Without the White gaze, these images did more than just showcase Asian men owning their erotic agency. More than that, it intimated that Asian men could be interested in each other, not relying on validation by the mainstream gay community. Though the message was specific to HIV prevention, the broader narrative was empowerment and autonomy.

The campaign also featured one image of Asian woman-woman inti-macy (figure 8.3). At this stage, the agency was still struggling with what women's programming could look like, but everyone agreed that the campaign could not focus on men only. In that image, two women held and looked longingly at each other, with one cupping the other's bare breast with her hand.

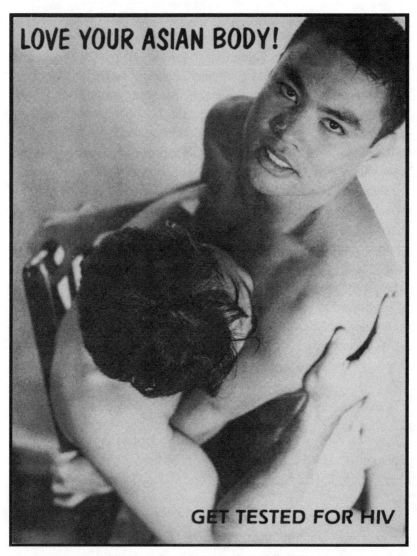

LOVE YOUR ASIAN BODY!

GET TESTED FOR HIV

FIGURE 8.2. Image from "Love Your Asian Body," APAIT's first social marketing campaign. Courtesy of APAIT, a division of Special Service for Groups, Inc.

The models were APAIT staff, volunteers, and clients. Unhei Kang, the first female staff at APAIT, was one of the women in the image; the other woman was a volunteer, an undergrad from UCLA. Eric Reyes, a volunteer at the time, was in at least two of the images. So was Keith Kasai, a client. The photoshoot took place at Ric's apartment, with just some plain bed sheets hanging in the background. "Doing it on the

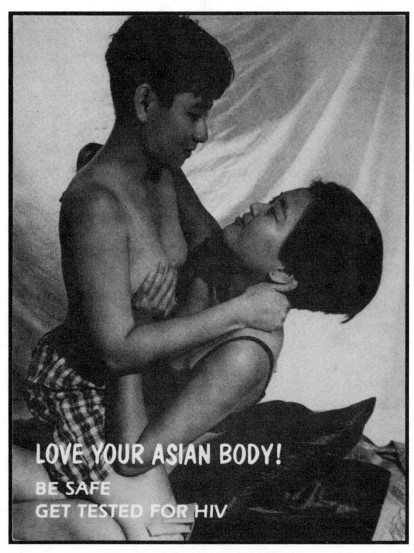

FIGURE 8.3. Image from "Love Your Asian Body," APAIT's first social marketing campaign. Courtesy of APAIT, a division of Special Service for Groups, Inc.

cheap" was a necessity from a limited budget, but the DIY vibe also reflected the young and emerging queer Asian community that the AIDS movement was fomenting.

In the essay "Communion," which he cowrote with Joël and others, Ric recounted looking for their ad in *Frontiers* and finding "page after page . . . filled with smiling white boys . . . with perfect bodies and airbrushed skin," the dominant icons of the gay beauty standard. When he finally came upon the "Love Your Asian Body" quarter-page ad in the back pages of the magazine, he noted, "It is the first time in Los Angeles we will see an API face on anything pertaining to AIDS on any significant scale. . . . I'm thinking perhaps one of the API kids we are trying to reach will stumble across an image of himself amongst all of this propaganda on the fabulous gay White life, then maybe it will spark something in him."

"It was a fun art project," said Joël of this first collective try at social marketing. "We got to call each other beautiful and took pictures of each other. It was kind of silly. It was definitely Asian American kids being Asian American kids. That's where the joy was. I'm so fond of the people."

Eric remembered it being a "very easy decision" to get involved as a model. He said, "I was their [Joël and Ric's] friend. We hung out all the time. When they asked, 'Do you want to do this?' I said, 'sure.' For me, it was, yeah, this makes perfect sense. Someone else said, 'I'll do it. It seems kind of fun.' This was serious stuff, but at the same time, there were giggling and funny moments. We're talking about male desire, and everyone in that room had different ideas and expressions of it. 'Stand there. Do this. Sit on his lap. Okay!' It was fun. Everyone was under thirty."

Unhei remembered similarly. When asked who came up with that image between her and another young woman, she said, "Some of it was planned out and some happened organically, after the camera started shooting." Caught up in the moment, no one was thinking about posterity. In our interview, I showed her reproductions of the "Love Your Asian Body" images to jog her memory. She said, "We were in our twenties. I'm forty-nine now, and when I look at these photos, I was like, 'What was I thinking?'" She smiled as she held a longer gaze at the photograph.

Eric said, "I used to have a folder of all these old API HIV/AIDS educational materials. They had these silhouette facials of an Asian person. They had bamboo or Chinese lanterns, some signifiers in a subtle way that said this is for APIs. We were very excited to be able to use colored paper, because color printing was way too expensive back then. They were so embarrassingly bad. They looked like things you see at a dentist's office. You can see how 'Love Your Asian Body' was so radical."

In using photographs of real people's faces, the new campaign was already a decisive break from these "old materials." According to Joël, the campaign deliberately traced its lineage to the cultural productions that emerged from the earlier years of AIDS activism. He said, "I saw 'Love Your Asian Body' in conversation with Gran Fury's Silence = Death or Read My Lips. At the time, it was pre-Facebook, pre-internet. It was about the power of the image." Gran Fury's "Read My Lips" graphic plastered the famous sloganeering of then President George H. W. Bush (as in "Read my lips: no new taxes.") against two men locking lips, in military uniforms, no less. The shock came from the unexpected juxtaposition of two things that didn't seem to belong together.

Alice Y. Hom, who later served on APAIT's community advisory board, was working as an intern at Highways Performance Space in 1991 under its founding codirector Tim Miller, and she saw firsthand how AIDS radicalized the local performance arts movement, too. Miller, a gay White man, was one of the NEA Four, solo artists whose National Endowment for the Arts grants were revoked in 1990 because of their works' sexual content. Highways had a reputation as the cutting-edge queer performance space and for its inclusion of people of color. APAIT staff members, like Joël, Noel, and Napoleon, had performed at Highways. Joël saw this space as "part of a whole engine of cultural production": "At the same time that 'Love Your Asian Body' was happening, I was producing shows with Luis Alfaro [an artist involved with Teatro Viva!, part of the Gay Men of Color Consortium] and Tim Miller at Highways to create a performative platform for gay Asian men and other queer people of color. In many ways, I was really alive in my arts, and the organizing was a natural part of that artistic production." Alice recalled, "Tim was a part of ACT UP. I was meeting people who were part of ACT UP. Later, I saw Justin Chin [who was HIV positive] take blood out of his own arm and then drink it. There's all this stuff happening on a cultural performance tip that I was becoming aware of when I worked at Highways. These artists . . . influenced what I was thinking about HIV/ADIS and what we need to do about it."

These reflections reminded me of Marlon Riggs, an African American filmmaker whose documentary *Tongues Untied* (1989) unabashedly celebrates Black gay bodies. The raw eroticism in his works took the negative sexual stereotypes of Black men head on, almost with a "And what?" attitude.

Or the independent film *The Living End* by Gregg Araki, which came out in 1992, the same year as the "Love Your Asian Body" campaign. In an interview in 2019, Araki described the nihilist road movie about two HIV-positive gay men who met after one of them killed a homophobic police officer, as "a diary for me. It was me spewing all of my dread about AIDS and the holocaust." When asked how the AIDS crisis informed the film, Araki said, "I hope that nobody ever had to go through what it was like to be young and gay and living in the late '80s, early '90s. It was a war zone, where you would feel like there's a target on your back and people are just dropped dead on the streets. It was nightmarish, surreal thing to live through. Also, it was so politicized. It was like, 'I'm literally being exterminated. I've been targeted for this genocide.'"

In works by gay male artists of color like Riggs and Araki, I inferred that the erotic of the most shocking kind went hand in hand with the anxiety about impending death. When death felt so near and almost inevitable, the erotic was defiant. As Joël added, "Consequently, the movement in gay communities of color followed suit with similar aesthetics. . . . All of a sudden a lot of these prevention campaigns were about Black-on-Black love, Latinos with Latinos. We followed suit, and we had cause to with all the rice queen syndrome."

Joël also credited the magazine *Lavender Godzilla* by the Gay Asian Pacific Alliance in San Francisco. He said, "*Lavender Godzilla* was a huge player in defining and creating gay Asian American culture, and a lot of us in the early movement wrote and published in there. There was an issue on smut, which at the time had a utopian element." By utopia, he meant the celebration of all kinds of sexual expressions, without being tethered by social conventions, like monogamy. He said, "I was so juiced by Queer Nation's radical broad sexuality. I didn't want our sexuality to disappear. If the mainstream or White supremacy would erase our sexuality, I compensated by being fucking hyper-sexual." Joël and other artists in the AIDS movement didn't want to see our desire buried under the fear of a deadly plague or watered down to win respect of others who otherwise wouldn't respect you. That kind of in-your-face sex-positivity drove Joël's own writing and performance arts, as it did for his peers. To him, "Love Your Asian Body" was one depot on this through-line. A self-described "porn hound" who had his eyes "burned out" from seeing "the nastiest things you can't imagine," Joël would continue this activism later by editing volumes of gay Asian erotica.

Though from an older generation, Dean also saw the need for the campaign. He said, "It was apropos for that time to focus on the actual Asian body. I don't think many Asians felt that they had a good body image. I know I didn't." Like his team, he felt that addressing that low self-esteem was a precondition to HIV prevention. He agreed that "it had to be provocative." The team kept pushing, and the only line Dean drew was "no pubic hair." Eric credits Dean for not standing in the way of the younger staff's initiative. He said, "[Dean] said yes to something when he had no idea what was going to happen. It takes a certain amount of strength to be able to take on that risk, because he was still responsible [as APAIT director]."

Some of the narrators recalled minor blowbacks. Ric said, "Some people thought we were just over the top, that it was too sexy. It was vulgar. And other people thought, 'Wow. What is this new generation of APIs? And what are they doing?' This is totally out of the mainstream and the traditional, be-polite, don't-make-waves kind of thing.'"

The only clear evidence I found of the campaign offending anyone was a letter I unearthed from one of Dean's old files he left behind after he retired. The envelope, with a return address of a "Donor Sperm Bank" in LA, included a clipped ad from *LN*. APAIT had taken out an ad there for a fundraiser, using the image from the "Love Your Asian Body" campaign featuring Unhei and another young woman. Written in longhand, the anonymous letter read, "Dear Staff, Many of us Gays have children and they say [see] what filthy dirty ad in the LN magazine. We will not support the Asian Pacific AID[S] Int. Team any more. We support the Aids funds all the time, but no more. Sincerely, Hundreds & Thousands of Gays."

To be honest, even the architects of the campaign had some skepticism about the effectiveness of the first APAIT social marketing effort. In "Communion," written shortly after the campaign took off, Ric wondered, "I'm not sure if this is the most effective route to go, but we have to begin somewhere. . . . They were reading the ads and they were talking about it. That was the point, wasn't it?" A few months later, when the county released new epidemiological data, Ric "suddenly felt personally responsible" for the continued rise of HIV infection in the Asian community in LA.

While extremely proud of the campaign, Joël recognized that it probably didn't make a dent with people who were at the highest risk:

> That epidemiological logic model is sound, right? Increase sense of self through this visual nationalism leads to lowering of HIV infection. That was the premise. That was also hyper-romantic. Who was it really for? We had our conversions of consciousness within our nucleus. We were learning together. But the people that we were targeting, a lot of them were newly arrived immigrants, not living a gay identified life. What the fuck would they care about "Love Your Asian Body"? I don't mean to be cynical, but that was for the funders on some level. Or for those who were already inclined towards that kind of social justice or community building. If you were already inclined, it was going to call to you.

Joël is not wrong. The "utopian" Asian-Asian desire put forth in the "Love Your Asian Body" campaign was far from the reality of many gay Asian men still subscribing to the White beauty myth. The campaign, as he said, "was in direct conflict with what the behavioral patterns were." Its most indelible impact probably was on me and my peers, college students coming of age in the relative safety and comfort of the higher education environment, critical of racism in the mainstream gay community, invigorated by ethnic and women's studies to embrace our marginalized identities, and looking for a community space to deepen this exploration. It was primarily this campaign that gave me the idea to work on this oral history, because at its heart, "Love Your Asian Body" was more than HIV prevention. For our generation, it was about offering a progressive alternative around which we could build a community and a movement. In those early years, APAIT was the place to be for queer Asian women and men inclined to this utopia where all of our selves were recognized and loved. We became volunteers and staff. Yes, the upstart organization depended on our labor for outreach, but that collective act of building this space also saved many of us, sharpened our political analysis, and gave us purpose. It was an intervention for us; we were the intervention.

And it didn't speak just to the men. Diep Tran, an undergrad at the time, could feel its effect all the way from the University of California at Riverside, miles (a couple of hours in traffic) away from any of the APAIT outreach venues. Having been drawn to APAIT partly by this campaign, she joined APAIT as a staff member in 1994. She said, "The ads were fantastic. They were just really sex-positive and graphic." She observed that later social marketing efforts moved toward conformity—the idea that "we look like everybody else, like United Colors of Benetton"—in order "to catch more people." She continued, "But in the beginning, it was just very specific. If you're a freak, a queer, you still deserve to live. It was very strong to me. Much more powerful than 'we're like everybody.'" This radical queerness drew Diep, me, and others like us to APAIT.

Dean was certain that the campaign raised the agency's profile with the funders and leaders of other AIDS service organizations. It put Asian faces on the AIDS epidemic, in very different ways that many hours of advocacy in a stuffy room couldn't. It showed to the powers that be that APAIT, though young, was a legitimate player in the growing field. Even through his reservations, Ric firmly believed that it laid the groundwork for APAIT to receive funding for direct services to people with HIV.

It wasn't just public health messages that were getting sexually explicit. Sex education, too, had begun to move away from the doom-and-gloom and the classroom recitation of basic facts. Shawn Griffin remembered that those early education modules were "just too judgmental, too preachy, and too black and white. You can't do this. You can't do that." They were also devoid of pleasure. He said, "It was layered with homophobia and heterosexism, as if they didn't care if two gay guys don't enjoy sex." Phill Wilson understood the shortcomings of this approach. He helped develop one of the earliest safer-sex curricula for Black gay men. He said, "We were going to continue to be sexually active. It was a nonstarter to think that people were not going to be sexual. So what were the things that we could do that would reduce the risk for HIV? How could you be sexually active and be sexually fulfilled without transferring bodily fluids?" Without mincing words, Phill called this workshop "Hot, Horny, and Healthy."

Prior to joining APAIT, Unhei went to a women's sex club in San Francisco with some friends. Safer Sex Sluts, a group that came out of

Mills College, was performing that night in a show supported by HIV-prevention funding. The group's name itself was enough to assure the audience that their safer-sex presentation would be anything but didactic and boring. Unhei recalled, "They were showing how you protect yourself with dental dams and cute little outfits. It was pretty explicit. Like simulated sex. On stage. At the same time, it was all very much like performance art. I was young. It was all very exciting, cool, and hip." Unhei didn't think it was just shock for shock's sake. "There was a lot of urgency back then," she said. "There were a lot of people who were dying. That's what it really came down to. I'm sorry, but it's a sexually transmitted disease. It was about how you get the word out."

APAIT was moving in the same direction. Joël said, "We had to develop the sex education for the next generations. The one we got was, . . . if you get this, you're dead. If you're gay, you're dead. I have to know there's hope in this. I have to know there's joy." Diep recalled having accumulated a collection of sex toys—dildoes, nipple clamps, and so forth—for her safer-sex demonstration and then having the chest of them stolen from her car trunk. While regretting the money that was lost in purchasing all that paraphernalia, she couldn't help but imagine the look on the thief's face when they opened the chest and realized what they had looted. She told this story to illustrate the importance of embracing the deviance when the old normal way of having sex was no longer safe or viable. The more gay sexuality was veering toward a "more legitimized . . . suburban bedroom situation," the more Joël "didn't shirk from a sexual storytelling" in HIV prevention. "Fuck that," he said, employing his catchphrase. "You got to think about Asian men doing nasty shit that's hot."

It was not your mother's sex education. Public health professionals call this the "harm reduction" approach, in stark contrast to the abstinence model which research consistently shows fails more than it works.

A closet academic who dropped out of college, Napoleon also took a scholarly approach. The framework he embraced was Paolo Freire's *Pedagogy of the Oppressed*. He explained, "You have to build people's connection with their own reality. These were usually young gay men we were talking to. We'd gyrate on stage. We did simulated sex acts to demonstrate." I don't know how many people have used Freire as a theoretical framework to free decolonized minds through public simulated sex. But AIDS did make for a strange reality in those days.

One time, Napoleon and his coworker Dredge Kang conducted a workshop at a community dance event. He said, "We did not have actual sex on stage, of course, but I guess it resembled enough that people thought it was. We were really nitty-gritty. We were like, 'If you want to make sure he's wearing a condom, try putting it on him yourself. And if he can't get hard for that, stimulate his nuts.' We were that detailed. We could still get away with it at that time, so we would take it to the edge." Napoleon recalled that the act got them into trouble with what he called "anti-pornography lesbians." While he understood the divide within the feminist movement about pornography, Napoleon, whose life could've been cut short any time by a slide in T-cells, responded, "You want AIDS education but you want no simulated sex whatsoever? What world do you live in? I had no time for people who were gonna blunt the necessity of honest sexual messages at that desperate time. I had no time for any of that."

The sexual explicitness of the "Love Your Asian Body" campaign and safer-sex education challenged the prevalent racial hierarchy that confined gay Asian men in either an invisible or subservient role. It was a frontrunner of an aesthetic tradition that would, a mere few years later, give rise to an emerging generation of young gay Asian visual artists. In his book *A View from the Bottom*, Nguyen Tan Hoang analyzed several documentary videos directed and produced by gay Asian men in the mid-1990s, including *Slanted Vision* by Ming-Yuen S. Ma and *7 Steps to Sticky Heaven* by Nguyen himself, both made in 1995. Nguyen wrote of these unapologetically graphic works, "A central component of the reeducation of desire for these films' intended gay Asian male audience is with a supposedly more empowering desire for other Asian men—that is, the conversion of 'potato queens' into 'sticky rice.' To paraphrase Marlon Riggs's famous dictum concerning gay black male identity, the political of gay Asian sticky rice desire can be summed up thus: 'Asian men loving Asian men is the revolutionary act.'"[1]

Nguyen further credited the AIDS movement in the queer Asian community as "another significant enabling context for the production of these works." From high art to pornography, and sometimes a blurred hybrid of experimental pornography, the artists were conscious of "a new queer Asian visibility" that was made possible by political organizing around HIV/AIDS. Nguyen wrote, "Throughout the 1980s and 1990s, community-based organizations dedicated to the education and prevention of AIDS adopted frank discussion of gay sex practices and the various risks for HIV and other sexually transmitted infections in safer-sex pamphlets along with multimedia campaigns such as flyers, posters, stickers, buttons, T-shirts and advertising at bus shelters, in subways, and on billboards . . . [They] utilized the codes and conventions of explicit, hard-core gay male pornography to eroticize safe sex in the service of the reeducation of desire."[2] The most self-conscious of the AIDS moment among the works that Nguyen discussed was Ma's *Slanted Vision*. In one segment, the film featured Napoleon reciting his poem about going on a pilgrimage to find a cure for AIDS, while in another, a safer-sex workshop disguised as a cooking demonstration— "a spoof of *Yan Can Cook*," Nguyen described it—as a Filipina drag queen prepared a chicken recipe (Chicken Fuk Yew), with "dildoes, zucchinis, dental dams, and a willing chicken, among other latex and organic ingredients." If AIDS activism didn't spark this new radical queer Asian consciousness, it had certainly enriched that conversation.

With more funding, APAIT continued to expand. Its social marketing campaigns began to cast a wider net to reach the broader Asian American community. As Diep suggested, even within a short time, the messages were becoming more mainstream.

CHAPTER 9

Do Your Job.
Piss Somebody Off.

BEFORE KAREN KIMURA JOINED THE ASIAN PACIFIC AIDS INTERvention Team (APAIT) in 1993, the South Bay (Torrance) native and a Cal State Long Beach graduate had been pursuing a master's degree in art at the State University of New York at Purchase. "I was only there for a couple of years, but I did take a class that changed my perceptions about AIDS," she said. "It was Kim Christenson's Political Economy of AIDS." A faculty in both economics and gender studies, Christenson's research on the AIDS crisis focused on the experiences of low-income women and on how resources were not as readily available to some populations. "She really brought that to light, and how New York responded," Karen continued. "I started going to ACT UP meetings. I went to the Gay Men's Health Crisis Center that was the first AIDS organization in the country. I got to meet people and learn firsthand about the epidemic. I did condom distribution and things like that." Her involvement with these pioneering organizations was "just at the surface level." She said, "My school wasn't in the city [SUNY Purchase is about thirty miles from Manhattan, close to the state's border with Connecticut]. And overall, the movement seemed to be . . . there was more involvement by White, gay male. . . . I went to my first March on Washington [March for Women's Lives in 1992]. I was over there for the Women's movement, so I was getting more politically active in different ways."

But the epidemic was creeping from the epicenter of gay New York. She added, "I was also teaching at the time. I was astonished that many of my students were shooting up heroin; some of them were gay or bisexual. It was beginning to hit closer to home."

When Karen came back to LA, her former classmates from Cal State Long Beach, Unhei Kang and Teri Osato, told her APAIT was hiring. Unhei was already a staff member, and Teri was a volunteer. Both were leaders in the local queer Asian women's community. Karen applied for the position managing the social marketing program Ric had started with "Love Your Asian Body." By then, he and Tracy Nako were moving to more client-centered work. Karen interviewed with Dean and Ric. Soon after, she became the second female staff member at the agency.

Karen suspected that the leadership had found her art background a transferable skill for the marketing work. Other skills were new to her, like working with ethnic media and developing an effective public health campaign. As a straight woman, she knew she needed help to craft messages that would engage that target population of gay Asian men or men who have sex with men (MSM). Ric was a mentor, not only because she inherited his program. His experience as someone living with HIV was valuable in making the work urgent and personal. But Karen also needed a day-to-day partner, and she knew she should find this person among the outreach team, who regularly interacted with people who needed to hear these prevention messages the most.

Around this time, also on the East Coast, a young Korean American college student was clocking quite a bit of field time in the AIDS movement. Even though Dredge Kang knew by the age of ten that he was attracted to men, it wasn't until he was nineteen, an undergrad at the University of Maryland at College Park, that he started thinking about the epidemic. He said, "I didn't have this automatic association between being gay and AIDS. Then once I started meeting other gay men, particularly older gay men, it became more real, since a lot of the older men were infected." Once he came out, he became what he called "a professional activist." His political interests were not limited to gay or AIDS causes. "Those were the days when abortion rights were a huge issue," Dredge said. "Well, these are the days again. We used to do something called 'clinic defense,' which is when we would create these paths for women who were seeking abortion services to be able to enter the clinic and not be harassed by people with signs and pictures of fetuses. Women's movement. People of color organizing. Issues around Palestine, too. It was a conglomeration of progressive causes that often share the same activists."

Off campus, a local Asians and Friends group in nearby Washington, DC, started an HIV-prevention program, and Dredge helped them "get the HIV testing off the ground." From there, he was recommended to the Korean Community Service Center, which had just received some HIV funding. Dredge said, "The director of that program called and asked me to work for them. There were two of us in the HIV program. I was doing the youth outreach. The other staff, a woman, focused on women, including massage parlor workers. Because of this job, I started going to conferences. National conferences often happened in DC, so everybody came to DC at some point. I met activists from all over the country. I remember meeting people like Joël Tan, Eric Reyes, Vince Crisostomo, Prescott Chow, and Steve Lew." (The last three were AIDS activists in the Bay Area.)

New AIDS funding gave Dredge Kang and other young gay men employment opportunities. Dredge dropped out of the school because he was so busy with his activism (he later returned to school and received his PhD in anthropology from Emory University in 2015). He was at Korean Community Services Center for about a year before he got his next offer that would take him to the West Coast.

He said, "I got a call from Joël Tan. He said that they had gotten new funding at APAIT and were interested in seeing if I wanted to apply. Joël wasn't the most subtle person. He said, 'We want you to come and work here,' and kind of offered me the job. I mailed in my résumé and cover letter. Then Dean Goishi called me on the phone, and we did an interview." The new funding came from the state of California to do outreach to MSM. The state funding complemented the outreach contract APAIT already had from the county, which was managed by Noel Alumit. "At the time, they had Filipinos and Japanese on staff. There were a lot of Chinese volunteers. So they were looking for somebody who was Korean because the Korean community in LA was large."

Dean saw (or heard) what Joël saw in Dredge and offered him the job officially. Dredge said, "It was at the time my dream job because it fit with where I was and what I wanted to do. In a sense, it was a way of being a professional 'gayasian' before gayasian-ness was a thing. I'd be working with the community I identified with. That was very important to me because I was still in that process of figuring out who I was."

With the job offer, Dredge left for LA in 1993. He had just turned twenty-two.

Because there had been another outreach program targeting the same population, Dredge and another new staff member, James Sakakura, had to find ways to distinguish themselves. Dredge explained:

> We experimented with different approaches. The agency had a long history of doing outreach at bars. We were always at Mugi's. It was a weekly stop. Then there was an explosion of one-night-a-week night clubs [for gay Asian men], like the Buddha Lounge, so we went to all those venues. The other program also went to bathhouses and sex clubs. So the gay venues were covered. James and I worked on more ethnic-specific venues. We were thinking where gay API men lived their lives in LA and who would have less access to the kind of information that we wanted to get across.

They went to less obvious outreach places like Filipino hair salons and Korean grocery stores and garment shops. Then he got a tip from Tracy Nako, who had heard that Asian trans people often congregated late at night at the Yukon Mining Company. Located in a strip mall on Santa Monica Boulevard, the twenty-four-hour diner in Hollywood was a haven for the transgender crowd until it closed in the early 2000s. Dredge said, "None of us had heard of this. One night, I went down just to check it out. There were a whole bunch of Asian trans people there, and Latino and African American [trans people] as well. We found out there was a club across the street that had a transgender night. This area was also a hub of trans sex workers in LA. We had never worked with the transgender population, so we started going every weekend to the Yukon Mining Company. I made that one of our new priorities, one of our regular outreach spots."

The new outreach spot prompted APAIT to hire its first transgender staff member, Darryl Arnau. As an outreach worker, the Yukon Mining Company became "one of her regular routines." Darryl's hiring "opened a whole new world," Dredge recalled. "We started doing transgender sensitivity trainings. We started working with other organizations and pushing transgender issues at a policy level. That was a time of possibilities. Everything was just growing."

When Karen came on board, she knew that to increase the awareness of the epidemic in the ethnic Asian communities, the social marketing campaigns had to reach a broader base than "Love Your Asian Body" had. "The population was so diverse and had so many needs," said Karen. "It's not like there was one method that was going to reach everybody. We would do a campaign for the more overtly gay identified, but then we would also do one that had more to do with families and community because we knew that being a part of the family or a community was a big part [for the target population]."

Yet with limited funding, she was mindful that APAIT might not be able to do it all. Karen asked, "What was the biggest bang for the buck?" There were two different kinds of campaigns. The first, like "Love Your Asian Body," featured images that were printed in LGBTQ publications or got passed around in bars in West Hollywood—what Karen called "the obviously gay targeted." Dredge and Karen came up with a new slogan called "Use Your Noodle," a follow-up to APAIT's first social marketing campaign to promote HIV testing. In Dredge, Karen found not only a thought partner for the next campaign, but also one of the campaign's models.

Dredge said, "The images were basically me and Jay [Williams, a biracial staff member of Japanese descent] playfully, semi-nakedly, feeding each other udon noodles. Use your noodle, like using your head, before engaging in risky practices." In retrospect, Dean thought the slogan, "Use Your Noodle," was so colloquial that most recent immigrants wouldn't understand it, or it would lose its nuances if translated into any Asian language. Also, Dredge acknowledged the same reservation that other staff had of the first campaign: "It played to the 'gayasian' way of thinking. It doesn't make sense otherwise."

"The early work was focused on self-esteem as the way to do HIV prevention," Dredge continued.

> That was this huge unspoken underlying theoretical framework that we all were using at the time . . . because of the stigma that people faced, both having HIV, as well as being gay and API, that we were so

undesirable as partners and things like that. Clearly our message was, the Asian body is worthwhile, that it deserves love. A lot of the activist work was very focused on reinstalling the value of being gay and Asian. People aren't going to protect themselves unless they love themselves. If you ask me now [laughs], I would say it's a mixed bag. Clearly it's important, but it's also not the only thing that needed to be emphasized. One of the contradictions of the epidemic is that places where gay men had the highest self-esteem were the places where gay men had the highest rates of infection. It's not just a matter of boosting self-esteem.

Napoleon Lustre, who was already living with HIV, also took issues with the self-esteem approach because it "just took too damn long." When I asked him whether these campaigns were cutting-edge, he responded, "It was and it wasn't. We co-opted the self-help language around loving yourself. I think you can do AIDS work without having to mine all that stuff, and you can still keep people uninfected without building up their fucking self-esteem. You can't wait. You have to save them now."

APAIT continued to experiment with social marketing messages that offered different and sometimes competing versions of what being an LGBTQ person in the Asian American community could mean. The aspirations of an LGBTQ Asian identity were anything but monolithic. In later years, Noel would assume the role of developing these campaigns. For his first try, he recruited "Asian go-go boys" for the photoshoot.

He said, "As far as I knew, no one [at APAIT] had done that. It was always our friends. I really wanted the gorgeous guys in the same way that AIDS Project Los Angeles or AIDS Healthcare Foundation was doing. They were putting out these gorgeous guys, including from the Latino and Black communities. Shirtless, handsome. I just saw these beautiful Asian guys in West Hollywood. I explained the concept: we're going to have gorgeous Asian guys in Speedos. I said, 'We're doing this photo shoot. Can you come and do this?'" Noel also met a professional photographer in one of his outreach named Wayne Shimabukuro, who agreed to take the photos for free. The photoshoot took place at the APAIT office. Noel humorously recalled that other staff "wanted to be in the room [to gawk at the models], even though they had nothing to do with it" (figure 9.1).

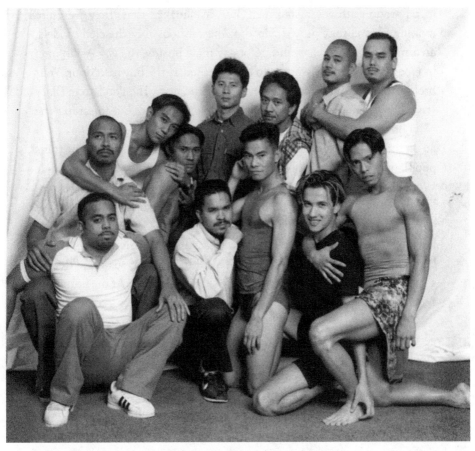

FIGURE 9.1. Male staff at APAIT, circa mid-1990s, mingled with Asian go-go boys during a photo shoot by Wayne Shimabukuro. Courtesy of APAIT, a division of Special Service for Groups, Inc.

He had another idea called "The New Boat People" that would feature "once again, gorgeous Asian guys kayaking, gorgeous Asian guys on a yacht, gorgeous Asian guys in a tub playing with a rubber ducky. It was always about gorgeous Asian guys." Noel thought it was a clever twist on Boat People. An aspiring actor at the time who had his share of being turned down for roles because of stereotypes of Asian men as asexual, Noel wanted this campaign to be a counternarrative. He said, "Looking back on it, I probably did it just for my own self-image. We wanted to see ourselves just as sexual beings, desirable beings." But when he worked with Nakatomi & Associates, a communications firm, and conducted a focus group with gay Asian men, he was shocked that "they were not looking for the sexy guy." Instead of these impossibly chiseled models, an almost unattainable standard of gay male beauty, the gay Asian men in Noel's focus group "wanted to be presented as the boy next door. Your brother. The ordinary college guy, trying his best. The good son. That's what they wanted to be seen as." Noel had no choice but to scrap "The New Boat People" idea.

In the mid-1990s, with Darryl on board, APAIT also targeted the trans population with its social marketing. Darryl came up with the "Bionic Woman" campaign. Posing as a model, Darryl is fully regaled in a strapless ball gown. A sparkling necklace hangs on her bare neck, right above her cleavage. Her left leg pushes through the dress's opening, revealing her high-heel. Around her, callout boxes point to various parts of her body, like price tags: "Nose Job: $4,000"; "Liposuction: $6,000"; "Reconstructed vagina: $15,000"; "Adams apple shaving; $1,500." At the bottom of the image is the message, "Protect that precious body! Use a condom."

Dredge, Darryl's supervisor, explained, "[These were] the kind of surgeries or procedures that people, if they're transitioning male to female, would go through. The message was, 'You've invested a lot in this body. You want to invest in its health, too. Take care of it.'" He actually had some reservations about it. He said, "I felt it was too commercially oriented, like you shouldn't care about your body just because you've put $25,000 in it. But it's the one that went through the process of community input." In the end, he deferred to Darryl and the trans community she had consulted.

After "Use Your Noodle," APAIT began to experiment with the second type of social marketing campaign that focused on the broader Asian American community. The images from either "Love Your Asian Body" or "Use Your Noodle" were more "overtly gay" than what the ethnic media would run. Whether it was homophobia or discomfort, Karen recalled, the images provoked such comments from some ethnic presses as "Are you sure this is what you want?" or "This does not really affect our community." These ethnic presses were crucial for broader AIDS education because they would reach those who were not already in the "WeHo life" and who were "not going to respond to the more overtly gay images." Reaching this MSM population was the holy grail of social marketing, the target audience that had been missed by the other gay-identified campaigns. It was also important to get the broader community to become more sympathetic so these MSM would feel less stigmatized about getting tested or seeking help. Karen persisted, and the ethnic presses usually relented. "A lot of times, it came down to the fact that we had money to pay for the ad," she said. "It's a business, and they would take the business."

Cultural and linguistic competence was Special Service for Group's (SSG) bread and butter. By 1993, SSG had established Pacific Asian Language Services (PALS), which closely worked with APAIT and its HIV-positive clients to provide interpretation at their medical appointments. Some PALS interpreters also helped APAIT translate social marketing messages in different languages. She said, "There was a lot of going back and forth. Like, 'Well, you're saying this, but that doesn't make sense in Thai.' Or, 'When you're saying this in English and you want to translate this in Cambodian'—or whatever language it was—'you had to change it so that it's not so in your face.' It was difficult, with me being English speaking only. I learned a tremendous amount."

The social marketing in each ethnic community sometimes took a decentralized approach. "We allowed the staff who were working with those communities to come up with a set of possibilities," Dredge said. "I don't remember all of them. They were often things like proverbs. There was one in Vietnamese, which was about how you wouldn't lie in a bed without checking for fleas first. Different kinds of sayings and proverbs from different groups that people might be more familiar with, that we thought would get across with monolingual [non-English speakers] in a more appropriate way."

APAIT staff also recognized that they probably needed a different kind of campaign than the ones that targeted gay men or MSM, one that targeted the broader immigrant community to reduce AIDS stigma. The in-house staff had been an incredible resource when the social marketing was focused on populations they knew intimately. To go broader would take expertise that even SSG didn't have. For instance, SSG did not write press releases or organize press conferences. They did not store a list of media contacts on a rolodex or a spreadsheet. Like most nonprofits, they did not have the bandwidth or resources to manage public relations. To run a social marketing campaign of APAIT's expanding ambitions, they needed to look outward. And they found someone—neither gay nor Asian, but willing to work cheap.

Robert Berger first heard about AIDS straight from the horse's mouth. On a flight back to his home in San Francisco in the early 1980s, he found himself sitting next to Dr. Anthony Fauci. Shortly after this encounter, in 1984, Dr. Fauci was appointed the director of National Institute of Allergy and Infectious Diseases, one of the research centers that make up the National Institutes of Health. From there, he made significant contributions to our understanding of AIDS and the virus that causes it. As the spokesperson of AIDS research under an administration (Reagan's) not especially sympathetic to people dying of AIDS, Fauci would initially be the target of many movement activists who did not think the government was doing enough. But he would prove to be one of their most even-keeled allies in the government. Robert met him on the plane just before he became the center of all this attention. "It was before [AIDS] was even named," Robert said. From Fauci, he got the firsthand account of the epidemic's projected path. It wasn't too many years later when he realized that what Fauci had told him was "spot on."

At the time, Robert was living a cozy but soulless life as an ad executive. In 1987, he moved to LA with the advertising agency he was working for. He got married and had two children. Now in his early thirties, none of these life events could quell his restlessness. "I started to become very disillusioned, disenchanted, with my work," He said. "I was pushing products that I didn't care about. I was very good at it, but it wasn't something that I got my fulfillment from. I got a decent paycheck and that was about it."

In the early 1990s, Robert "decided to go another path." He launched a business with his then-wife, Dr. Eileen Chun, an internist with a private practice. Focusing on social marketing in public health, the new company, Healthier Solutions, "would be an interesting combination of my marketing and communications skills and her medical and public health insights. It was a for-profit company, but it wasn't motivated primarily by profit. I was going into an area where there weren't the multimillion-dollar budgets I was used to in advertising." Robert started to reach out to diverse communities in LA and volunteer with organizations that served African Americans, Latinos, or Asian Americans. At one time, he served as the vice president of the Asian American Advertising and Public Relations Alliance. While serving as a cochair for the Asian Pacific American Heritage Month, he met Herb and Naomi at SSG. (The Heritage Month was an initiative from the mayor's office, but SSG handled its fiscal and administrative functions.)

SSG was expanding. In a few more years, they (along with APAIT) would move from their dingy office in the Westlake neighborhood (just west of downtown LA) to the Standard Oil Building, an officially registered historic monument just blocks from the Los Angeles Convention Center and what would become the Staples Center before the end of the millennium. In the 1990s, SSG didn't have a staff dedicated to public relations. In fact, while their programs were beloved by the local communities they served, most people didn't know what SSG, the parent company, was, and Herb had been happy to stay out of the spotlight and let the individual divisions shine. The growth demanded more coherent branding at the very least. Recognizing Robert's expertise, Herb connected him to some of the SSG divisions. For a while, Robert worked with the Homeless Outreach Project (at the time serving mostly African Americans in South LA) and the Asian Pacific Counseling and Treatment Center, both SSG stalwart divisions. The diversity of issues and target populations was just what Robert's new company needed to cut their teeth on. "What really took off in a wonderful way," he said, "was the relationship with APAIT. I found Dean and the whole staff very welcoming and open. Once there was trust built and they knew that I was doing this for the right reason, we worked together to tell their story through marketing and help raise the profile and reach of the organization."

About a decade after randomly meeting Dr. Fauci on a plane and hearing about the impending epidemic, working with APAIT seemed almost "fateful" to Robert. Together, Robert and APAIT launched the Facing HIV and AIDS campaign. The campaign wasn't focused on changing people's behavior (like getting tested or engaging in safer sex) as much as changing their minds. Drawing on his experience of promoting breast cancer awareness for the state of California, he saw a parallel in AIDS. "We were dealing with a lack of understanding and appreciation that AIDS was something that the community needed to be aware of, to be supportive of, and that there were services available for it," he said. "I faced this in my breast-cancer work. People need to identify and say, 'There's someone like me or from my community dealing with the issue.' Otherwise, there's denial. 'It's not us. It's not our issue.' The Facing HIV and AIDS campaign was designed, literally, to put an Asian face on the issue."

Well, more than one Asian face. There were a dozen people involved in this campaign, with their images plastered on billboards and bus benches in neighborhoods with a high concentration of Asian immigrants, like the San Gabriel Valley, Chinatown, and Koreatown, as well as in the ethnic presses. Robert assembled a panoramic lineup of Asian Americans, young and old, male and female, from different ethnic groups, sitting in two rows, like a portrait of a large family. Karen described the photo as "not so overtly gay"—so that people wouldn't dismiss the message out of hand. The caption read, "Two of Us Are HIV Positive," and in smaller print, "You Do Not Have to Face HIV and AIDS Alone." The campaign challenged commonly held assumptions about people living with HIV. You can't tell who has HIV by looking at a person. They could be your grandfather, your sister, your child, your neighbor; or as Robert said, someone you could identify with in your community, so that you couldn't deny AIDS's impact around you. He said, "It made people ask, 'Which two [in the photo have HIV]?' Really, the answer is, it could be anyone."

Even with a professional behind the scenes, the campaign was looking for "ordinary people" to pose for the photoshoot. Naomi Kageyama said, "We were just grabbing people around the office and making sure we have those who were gay and straight, to show the community that's very diverse, and multiple generations. Even Herb had his daughter in the picture." Naomi was part of the lineup as well. She had to think about the ramifications of being so visibly implicated with HIV. She said, "I'm still part of that generation that doesn't make waves. You're polite and don't shout to make yourself known. And wow, I'm going to be on a billboard. I had to grapple a little bit internally. Like, am I comfortable with this? I had family and friends who didn't understand my job. I had to get over my shyness. Beyond shyness, I had to get ready to boldly state this is my profession, this is what I do to empower others."

The use of everyday people was not a cost factor but was actually consistent with Robert's approach to the campaign. He said, "I'm a stickler on keeping things real. I don't hire actors. It's not a casting call for an Advil ad. I can't think of a situation where we said, 'No, we can't use you.'

The only thing that guided us at the time was, 'Well, we need someone who's young, someone who's older.' We wanted to be inclusive." The agency was actually very deliberate in featuring many women in the photo. Infection rates among women of color were just starting to go up in a way that would soon shatter the myth that AIDS was a gay man's disease. But in the early 1990s, Robert thought APAIT was "ahead of the curve" in terms of gender parity. He said, "At that time, we didn't have the data to back it up, but we knew it was the right thing to do."

Because these weren't actors, Robert conducted media training with the grassroots models before the photoshoot. He said, "We talked about potential issues that might come up to make sure that folks are comfortable." The photographer he hired, however, was anything but DIY. Don Farber was an award-winning photographer who had worked with the Dalai Lama, among others.

On the day the billboard was unveiled, Robert drove to Koreatown. The former advertising executive was nervous about how well the campaign would be received. "It was the first Asian-language, multimedia campaign in LA County, if not the country," he recalled. "There wasn't 'Let's do what they did.' There was no 'they.'" At the intersection of Olympic Boulevard and Western Avenue, above a car dealership, Robert found the billboard (figure 9.2). "That was a highly visible location. A lot of traffic. I parked my car, and I was observing people that were stopping at the light. They would do a double take, or even a triple take."

Despite the campaign's being "not so overtly gay," the publicity generated backlash in the Asian American community. The negative comments were more swift and intense from the Chinese community, said Dean. A Chinese American attorney asked him, "Why are you putting this HIV infection in the middle of our community? We don't have it. We'll never have it." Robert recalled several churches being upset. Noel remembered that staff got "a call from a pastor saying that [the billboard] was inappropriate." This pastor in the San Gabriel Valley "wanted it to come down because he said we were bringing the disease into the community," said Heng, who by that time was running PALS for Health and provided the translation for the campaign. Noel also recalled, "Unhei forward[ed] a call to all of us with a death threat, saying, 'You don't deserve to live.' It was just this wake-up call that there were people who just did not like us."

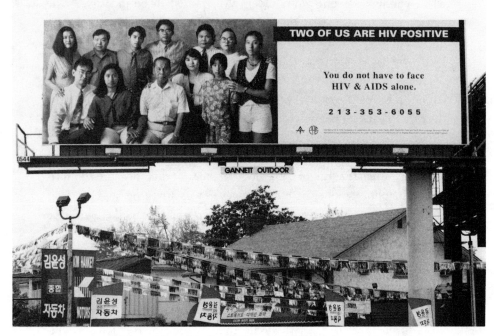

FIGURE 9.2. Billboard from "Facing HIV and AIDS" social marketing campaign above a car dealership in LA's Koreatown. Courtesy of Robert Berger.

The pushback only confirmed for Robert and others that the campaign was working. He said, "If you're not pissing somebody off, you're not really doing your job. I did a lot of public policy work on tobacco. A lot of smokers were upset and threatened my life. I had to be escorted by police out of city council meetings a few times. The reality is, if you're successful in a campaign like this, not everyone's gonna be happy. It comes with the territory."

Heng agreed. "It ruffled some feathers in the community, but that was good, because it meant that people were looking at it." Naomi felt even more bluntly: "There are always going to be assholes. At some point, we would laugh it off. Well, it's good that it gets people talking."

The billboards were the cornerstone of an umbrella campaign. Leveraging his professional relationships, Robert worked with APAIT staff, like Karen, on a media blitz. He organized press events that featured both APAIT staff who were HIV positive and medical experts (including his wife at the time) as spokespeople, targeting all media formats—newspapers, radio, and television—reaching across diverse ethnic communities. Some of the English-language press targeting these communities, like the *Rafu Shimpo* (Japanese) and *TM Herald Weekly* (Filipino), covered these stories enthusiastically and sympathetically. Robert also remembered the publisher of *Siam Media News*, a Thai paper, "embraced the issue and was always there for us." Both the Filipino and Thai communities were disproportionately affected by the epidemic. Also, some of the papers in the smaller ethnic communities were limited in staffing and resources and were so neglected by the mainstream that they were starving for ready-made content. APAIT also greased the wheel by purchasing ads in return. "It wasn't a big budget," Robert said. "But small budget can go pretty far in some of these media outlets."

The campaign won awards and recognition from both the advertising industry and the nonprofit sector, like the National Association of Social Workers. In 1995, APAIT took home the Horizon Award for a nonprofit program from Western International Media, "a big media outfit" that had been Robert's partner on ad distribution. With its Facing HIV and AIDS campaign, APAIT began to penetrate the more mainstream segments of the Asian ethnic communities. That influence would grow with the help of allies, particularly Asian American celebrities and artists, many of whom were straight but had seen how the epidemic took the lives of colleagues and devastated their industries.

While ostensibly an advocacy for HIV/AIDS, such work also elevated the discussion about sexuality in the immigrant communities and thrust many LGBTQ AIDS activists onto the leadership stage. With APAIT's profile raised, the local ethnic media in immigrant communities began to approach its staff for stories. The editor at *KoreAm Journal*, for instance, contacted Dredge because they were working on an issue on AIDS and LGBTQ Koreans. Dredge said, "The editor was known to be a pretty progressive guy. My first response was, those are two separate issues. So you need to do different issues, one on LGBT and another on HIV/AIDS, but we're not going to mix the two. They agreed to do that." The journal published a "queer issue" on August 1993, and the "HIV/AIDS issue" three months later. Dredge and Unhei appeared on the cover of the queer issue, along with two UCLA students. *KoreAm Journal* would become a much glossier magazine, but in 1993, Dredge described it as a bimonthly newsprint. Yet the fact that a mainstream Korean press outlet was willing to take on these taboo subjects was a big deal, even if *KoreAm Journal*, published in English, served mostly a younger, more assimilated Korean American readership. "They got a lot of attention," Dredge continued. "I still see those issues of *KoreAm* floating around."

After those issues came out, other Korean media followed suit, including *Korea Times* and local radio programs. A Korean-language television program on local cable, *LA Seoul*, asked Dredge and others at APAIT to put together an LGBTQ panel. Dredge recalled, "It was back in those pre-internet days. People watched TV together. There was a lot more exposure for [a local cable] show. That show was broadcast in Korean, so it made a huge splash among the monolingual community. There were four of us on the show. Except for one person, the other three of us were all primarily English speakers. When we responded in English, they would do simultaneous interpretation." Language became a compromise for who could be a spokesperson for the community. Many LGBTQ Koreans who could speak Korean fluently did not want to be out on a show that many in the community watched. Dredge explained, "We decided early on that we wouldn't have anybody with a brown paper bag over their head. That was what people were used to, that if you were queer, you had to be ashamed, and you couldn't show yourself. We could've had more people who were fluent in Korean on the show, but the flip side was that it would be this reinforcement of the closet. We didn't want to portray that."

Instead, the mostly English-speaking panelists exuded confidence on the show. One of Dredge's friends—who was not out to his family—watched the show with his mother. Dredge remembered him "distinctly saying that his mom commented that when I was talking about being gay, I said it without any shame. She thought it was shocking. But that was the point."

Although Dredge and his colleagues insisted that queerness and HIV/AIDS were two separate issues, there was no question that raising the profile of one highlighted the other. The normalization of non-heteronormative sexualities was essential in encouraging people living with HIV in these ethnic communities to come out and seek help. In some cases, coping with the virus also meant possibly reconciling with their birth families. By advocating for one of the most stigmatized populations in our communities, AIDS activists began to change attitudes toward LGBTQ people, regardless of their HIV status. It allowed them to come home.

CHAPTER 10

Interpreters of Maladies

ASIAN PACIFIC AIDS INTERVENTION TEAM'S (APAIT'S) INITIAL funding focused on HIV prevention: outreach, education, social marketing. With their brand of cultural and linguistic competence, they could reach out to Asian men who have sex with men (MSM) like nobody's business. When it came to the bigger pot of money for client services, APAIT still hadn't established a track record of serving people living with HIV to compete with the larger AIDS service organizations. Even without funding early on, Ric Parish and Sally Jue ran a support group in Ric's apartment for Asians living with HIV. Her social work expertise complemented his lived experience with the virus.

Napoleon Lustre, another HIV-positive member of the staff, took over the support group in the mid-1990s. He ran it like a "networking social" because Asians didn't "have the practice in going to support group of any sort." He said, "We were flying by the seat of our pants. We did it like the natural, organic way. You want to get together? We'll have a party. We're APIs [Asian Pacific Islanders]. We must have food. It was instinctive, the way we understood ourselves culturally. There were maybe five of us that first attended."

The group included his coworker at APAIT, James Sakakura, whose passing a couple of years later would have a huge impact on the entire staff. "There was this younger man, really good-looking and muscular, like a West Hollywood clone but Asian," Napoleon continued. "He was someone I'd never met before. We were a range of ages, from twenties to fifties. I think I was the youngest one there. We developed a bond very quickly." The only other survivor from this original group was Gil Mangaoang, whom Napoleon quickly discovered was "someone majorly important in the community that goes back to the late sixties, an experienced and effective organizer." That, and their shared Filipino heritage, made them "gravitate to each other." Gil spoke of the importance of having Asian-specific support groups:

> I didn't like the support groups at APLA [AIDS Project Los Angeles]. It was more, well, we have support groups and they were for everybody of every culture. A lot of the attitudes of APLA reflected, I think, the hierarchy of the gay movement: basically white-oriented, middle class kind of values, supposedly not racist. As large as that organization was—remember when they had that big monstrosity there on Vine Street?—there were not many people of color. . . . They wouldn't understand and be able to interact with me and appreciate the isolation that [I felt as] a man from a Filipino background. . . . No, I knew something better was out there. When I went to APAIT . . . well, there were Filipino, Chinese, Vietnamese, also Thai. Different Asian peoples living with HIV, at different stages. I felt that there was that commonality of how difficult it is to disclose within the Asian culture, and all the discriminatory aspects that come into play.

Napoleon added, "The support group would go on for a while, but it took a while to build into a good solid number. Those were the days when people went to support group to have support dying. There was this unspoken contract that we would take care of the ones that were getting ill, and hope that someone would be there when it was your turn."

Another strategy to support HIV-positive clients was to lean on the army of volunteers APAIT had trained, including many young LGBTQ Asian Americans who were hungry for a friendly space where they could have a hand in shaping a community they could claim. Connie Wong, whose leadership at the Los Angeles Asian Pacific Islander Sisters overlapped her time on the community advisory board at APAIT, volunteered for the APAIT's buddy program. She was paired up with Karen Kimura to be a buddy to a woman client.

A buddy tried to reduce the isolation and depression of someone living with HIV by providing company in social outings, medical appointments, or general errand running. Sometimes, a buddy even helped out with a house chore or two. Most AIDS service organizations do not have buddy programs anymore because people living with HIV nowadays can live healthy and independent lives. But in those early days of "everybody does everything," it was not uncommon for staff like Karen to take on volunteer functions, even if they were not part of their job descriptions, to learn more about the epidemic's impact on the community. A buddy might be a rare contact a person living with HIV had in any given week. In many cases, people who needed buddies were shut-ins who knew the best years of their lives were behind them and that there probably wouldn't be that many years ahead of them. Even when they accepted help, they might not be in the most pleasant of moods.

Connie described her experience with this APAIT client, a Thai woman, being very challenging. "She complained about almost everything," Connie said. "I'm not sure she was angry because of HIV/AIDS or if she was just an angry person. She was divorced, and she didn't seem to have very many friends. Karen and I were sitting with her at lunch or dinner, and she was always angry about something." Connie knew that her job was "just to listen," but at times it became "very difficult."

Karen added, "She was visiting Thailand one time and got sick over there. She had to get a blood transfusion, and that's how she got infected. She thought it was her fault. She had a lot of regrets because she wanted to have children. That was difficult for her." Neither Karen nor Connie was clear if HIV infection was the reason for her divorce. Connie remembered meeting the ex-husband and thinking that "he was always around in the picture" and generally supportive, though Karen had no recollection of the man. Karen echoed Connie's assessment of this woman's isolation. Karen said, "She did not find support in her community. She lived in Monterey Park. I don't think she was out in that community with her status. APAIT really became her family. She had tried [the antiretroviral medication] AZT and different drugs, and they would just make her really sick. Towards the end, she was trying to balance it out with more of the holistic or herbal medicines. She loved to talk. She loved food, too, and we'd go out to eat."

Connie was in the buddy relationship for about two years before the client's health "slowly went downhill." She was in the hospital briefly before she died. Both Connie and Karen attended the funeral. Connie remembered that her body was cremated. Karen said that the funeral was organized by the church the woman attended, but "it wasn't explained that she had died of AIDS . . . because I don't think she wanted that." Karen admitted that the accumulation of this and other clients' deaths "ended up really taking its tolls over the years." You can't talk about the AIDS movement without talking about grief. As the agency began to expand its portfolio of client services, grief became inevitable and at times debilitating for staff.

Even with support groups and a buddy program, APAIT staff knew their clients needed services that they weren't providing yet in those early years, such as primary care, mental health counseling, and housing. Initially, they would connect these clients to existing programs in other organizations. What they found (and their referral partners recognized) was that, by providing consistent social and emotional support, a connection with APAIT, these clients would be more likely to keep their appointments and be compliant with their treatment plans. "There were unique things about Asians [that needed to be considered] in order to be successful in providing any services to those individuals," Dean explained. "It wasn't just about giving you housing or giving you food. It was, how could that person navigate through the system and still feel good about himself? Because if you didn't feel good about yourself, you were going to die very quickly. We made sure the cultural issues were addressed."

The first success APAIT had in accessing client services dollars was case management. A case manager assesses the holistic needs of a client, helps them access services that they need and are eligible for, makes sure the client has the wherewithal to stay on their plan, and advocates for the client when necessary. When the client misses an appointment, a case manager tries to find out why and get them back on track. Because most HIV-positive clients need a plethora of services from multiple agencies, a case manager is the nexus of all the service providers they come in contact with. Case management is what keeps them healthy between appointments.

Tracy Nako became the first case manager at APAIT in 1993. He said, "It started off very slow and small. This was something new in the Asian Pacific Islander community and it was very difficult to get clients to come in for case management. We found a lot of the clients because we were providing culturally relevant education and services to the Asian community. We were also getting referrals from the County-USC hospital and nonprofit organizations like the Gay and Lesbian Community Center." When these providers encountered an Asian client with HIV, especially if they were an immigrant with limited English proficiency, they knew having APAIT as a case management partner increased the likelihood of their staying on their treatment.

Tracy remembered having about sixteen or seventeen clients in the first year, short of the goal of twenty-five. "There were quite a few immigrants, and they were not identified as gay or bisexual. I had one woman client and a few straight men. I was surprised by how many immigrants were in the case management program that first year, and from all the different ethnic groups, Thai, Cambodian and Vietnamese, for example. And people lived all over the county. What was unique about the APAIT program was that I would go to people's homes in order to protect their privacy. I drove to Rosemead and the South Bay, all over the place, racking up the miles."

A monolingual English speaker, Tracy needed interpreters from APAIT's sister program, Pacific Asian Language Services (PALS), to work with many of these clients. They would accompany Tracy to a client's home or their medical appointments. From his observations, Tracy thought the language barrier was huge, and it often made a difference between a client seeking help or not. He explained, "There was so much marginalization with immigrants, especially if you were a gay immigrant. I rarely met family members. I'm sure they felt the stigma of being gay or having HIV, and the community was in denial that we had a huge problem of HIV or drug abuse." The stigma already made it hard for someone to come forward and ask for help. Having someone who spoke the same language and didn't act as if the client was a pariah made it easier for them to keep coming back for services.

Heng Foong was running PALS by the time Tracy came on board to APAIT. By then, PALS had been providing a one-day training to interpreters in different Asian languages on AIDS. It wasn't as easy as just finding people with the right language skill. "I was being very mindful that the people I recruited had to have that sensitivity and awareness," Heng said. "I remember this one woman applying to be a Korean interpreter. She was probably in her forties. I observed her at work. She treated this poor man with such disdain. She couldn't even say the word AIDS. I think she had some discomfort with the fact that the client was a gay man, and with the disease itself, which didn't show up during the HIV/AIDS 101 orientation. How do you pick the right person, back then when interpreting wasn't even thought of? There was no certification." Heng had to dismiss the interpreter. A few years later, she and her staff developed a weeklong training—much longer than the one-day orientation—with a final exam that candidates had to pass in order to become a PALS interpreter.

There was a reliable supply of PALS interpreters for Japanese, Korean, Thai, and a few dialects of Chinese. For a brief time in the late 1990s, I was a Cantonese interpreter. Heng said that "they were a constant presence at APAIT." Because of the linguistic diversity of the Asian immigrant populations, however, PALS and APAIT sometimes had a hard time finding a match for a client, especially from the smaller ethnic communities.

Once, Tracy had gone to Heng about a new client who spoke a language he didn't recognize. When they got on the phone together, Heng realized that she "understood a little bit of what he was saying." An immigrant from Malaysia, Heng recognized that the man spoke Indonesian. Without an Indonesian interpreter on PALS's roster of consultants, Heng's Malay was not ideal but "close enough."

As the man's interpreter, Heng now found herself in the shoes of her consultants and it gave her new insights about Asian immigrants living with HIV. "I remember going with Tracy to 5P21 [the AIDS ward at the County-USC hospital] and sitting there with this man who had both TB [tuberculosis] and HIV. He was being kicked out of his house because his roommates were afraid to use the bathroom after he used it. . . . I saw Tracy grabbing a roll of toilet paper from the Standard Oil Building [where the APAIT and PALS offices were located] to give it to him while he was staying at the Morrison Hotel down the street." Morrison Hotel, the namesake for an album by The Doors in the 1970s, had served as low-income housing for that part of Downtown LA until 2008. Heng continued, "That was how quickly he got kicked out of his house, and what APAIT needed to do to get him care. He was really sick. It made me appreciate what case managers like Tracy did at APAIT."

APAIT began to step up its programming for HIV-positive clients, making it easier for Tracy to retain them in his caseload. Besides the support groups and buddy program, the agency also started a dayroom in 1994 where clients could drop in every Wednesday, partake in different activities, and socialize with each other. Pauline Kamiyama, hired as an emotional support coordinator, ran the dayroom. The key ingredient, she said, was food. "Food brings everyone together. It brings out all these cultural memories, like cooking or eating with loved ones." She remembered picking up food donated by Asian restaurants in North Hollywood and Los Feliz. "We played games like cards and mahjongg. If you didn't know mahjongg, we'd teach you." She fondly recalled a client, Johnny, a fashion designer, who led a drawing class. "Johnny always came to the dayroom in fabulous clothes, but his apartment was a total chaos." A volunteer who was a professional photographer offered a workshop with a Polaroid camera. "He asked the clients to pose with happy faces, sad faces, just a range of emotions. As the photos were developing in front of them, they would have a discussion about their emotions right there. It was a non-threatening way to talk." Even just the act of sharing a meal could lead to personal revelations. Without forcing a conversation, the clients would discuss "fear of dying, being ashamed, being estranged from family, how to talk to family members." "We rarely sat in a circle," Pauline said. "Yet all these social activities were group therapy without being group therapy."

Pauline said that the clients who came to the dayroom were mostly gay men or MSM, at least initially, from a variety of ethnic groups. "They all spoke some English, some better than others." I told Pauline that I found it remarkable that neither language nor culture had prevented the pan-ethnic bonding. They were committed to each other. Pauline remembered a client, suffering from non-stop diarrhea because of his AIDS medication, who "still managed to come to the dayroom because it was that important to him." It had to be about more than a free lunch. "It helped to have James and Ric there. It was really empowering for the clients to see such strong gay Asian men who were HIV positive in the organization." Other client services staff, like Tracy, also attended the dayroom regularly to build relationships with the clients and provide support when the clients were ready for individual services.

A Vietnamese American client sent a testimonial letter to Dean in 1999:

> I was diagnosed HIV positive in 1992. . . . I was miserable, worried and lonely. I was totally confused and did not know which direction to go. It was then during this time that I was referred to Asian Pacific AIDS Intervention Team. Because I am Asian, I wanted to meet other Asians who have the same problems I have. It was 1994 when I started attending the Wednesday dayroom activities. The more I attended and participated with the various activities, such as small group discussion, one-on-one client and staff interactions, outings, seminars, etc., I developed trust and self-esteem and really felt that I found a home where I can be myself. It is very uplifting and empowering to be with other Asians because we all seem to have the same kind of sensitivity about personal issues especially as a PWA. . . . Today I am a completely different person—full of positive attitude about the future, enjoying good-quality life to its fullest each day and sharing my life experiences to others.

Some of APAIT's advocacy at the time was to justify these "loosely structured" activities—"come hang out and maybe talk if you want to"—as not just alternatives to conventional mental health interventions, but actually more effective ones for Asians. In 1994, APAIT contracted a consulting group to conduct a focus group with its clients. The consultants found that "for new immigrants, you have to have some kind of concrete assistance. Counseling doesn't mean anything to them. . . . As far as AIDS Program Office [LA County funder] is concerned, a game of mahjongg is not a support group, but that may be the best support group for some of our clients. We have to be creative in finding ways to describe and justify what we do to funders."

Whether it was a free lunch or mahjongg, the dayroom was more culturally appealing to many clients than support groups because, as Tracy said, "support groups are not like an Asian thing, but more of a mainstream model." In the initial years, the constellation of these programs meeting different needs in their clientele allowed a potential client to enter the agency through different doors and the agency to keep them close. This "synergy," as Tracy called it, allowed him to keep up with his clients. If he was concerned about a case management client, he could talk to the staff running the dayroom, and vice versa. After his first year, Tracy easily met the case management program's yearly target goal.

From the beginning, cultural and linguistic competence justified APAIT's niche in the Asian immigrant communities. Working with PALS interpreters made that case even more convincing. But cultural and linguistic competence wasn't just about a one-to-one match of cultural backgrounds between a client and a provider. As in the story Heng shared about the Indonesian client, that match wasn't always possible. APAIT's experience in serving HIV-positive clients revealed some nuances about our understanding of cultural competence. Tracy noticed that APAIT attracted more of the immigrant clientele, even though its staff were fairly assimilated. "That was the surprising thing for me," said Tracy. "I think the American-born gay Asians could be part of the bigger, mainstream organizations, like APLA." Many immigrant clients shunned going to community-based organizations in their respective ethnic community, because of their fear of exposure and judgment. However, a pan-ethnic agency, like APAIT, not embedded in any specific ethnic enclaves conferred an interesting insider-outsider status on the organization. Even if staff didn't speak a specific language, the agency was "Asian enough" for immigrant clients to still feel comfortable going and seeking help, but not so familiar that they would worry about other people in their ethnic community finding out they were HIV positive.

Once it got going, APAIT's scope of services for HIV-positive clients continued to grow. An epidemic without modern precedence, AIDS required some innovation in public health. Treatment advocacy was one of those innovations, one for which APAIT played a key and pioneering role. Through the AIDS commission, LA County had set up fairly rigid funding service categories. Treatment advocacy became another battle-front where Asian American AIDS activists forced the burgeoning AIDS bureaucracy to adjust.

CHAPTER 11

We Want a New Drug

ALMOST SEVEN YEARS INTO THE EPIDEMIC, THE FDA APPROVED the first drug to treat AIDS in the US. Developed in the 1960s, azido-thymidine, or AZT, had been an anti-cancer drug that showed little promise but a lot of side effects. In the simplest terms, AZT inhibits HIV from replicating itself, but healthy cells are the collateral damage. AZT is chemotherapy in the form of a swallowable drug. Scientists called AZT a kind of "nuke"—a shorthand for "nucleoside analogue"—though the reference to a "nuclear option" or the similar effect a nuclear radiation has on someone was also apt. Of the four Asian American activists I interviewed who are HIV positive, none had taken AZT in those early years. In fact, every one of these activists independently told me that they suspected they were still alive because they didn't take AZT when it was the only option. Gil Mangaonang called AZT "a killer . . . a poison essentially." After seeing how others writhed under the drug in the late 1980s, Ric Parish was determined to stay "treatment naïve" so that his body wouldn't develop any resistance to better therapies that would come along later. In a controversial article in *SPIN,* published in 1989, reporter Celia Farber found that "the last surviving patient from the original AZT trial . . . died recently. When he died, he had been on AZT for three and one-half years. The longest surviving AIDS patient overall, not on AZT, has lived for eight and one-half years." Other studies did not necessarily show AZT to be useless, but its effects were short-lived, as the virus could easily mutate and become resistant to the drug. When little else showed promise in those early years of the epidemic, AZT was a Hail Mary drug.[1]

The FDA approval of the first AIDS drug was actually fast-tracked. A drug approval usually took eight to ten years and required at least three double-blind human trials. AZT was approved after one, and that one trial lasted only sixteen weeks, well short of the typical six months most trials took to determine both the drug's effectiveness and safety. The findings from this quick study were later found to be premature or even invalid. The whole process to get AZT from the laboratory to the market took all of twenty months.

The initial pricing of the drug was also controversial. Though AZT was not the silver bullet that everyone was hoping for, it was still, as Gil described, "the straw people grasped because it was the only thing that was offered during that time." But the ability to even grasp this first and only straw was not afforded equally for everyone. A year's worth of AZT treatment cost about $8,000 in 1987—$18,000 in 2021 dollars—a sum that many who were uninsured could not afford. In actuality, AIDS treatment was even more costly than that, as the side effects of AZT could be alleviated only by other drugs or therapies. The cost of treatment also made it harder for people with HIV to obtain health insurance. In the age of insurance denial for preexisting conditions, the health insurance industry found new ways to avoid not only people who were tested positive for HIV, but also those they considered high risk. A 1989 article in the *New York Times* reported that to "limit risk," coverage was sometimes denied to "men who are not married or who have jobs that are stereotypically associated with gay and bisexual men, like hairdressing."[2]

In 1987, the year that AZT was approved, the Centers for Disease Control and Prevention estimated that there were over five thousand deaths from AIDS complications. About 562,000 people were living with HIV, of which 84,800 were new infections that year. The public was becoming more aware of the epidemic, an awareness that fanned both paranoia and sympathy. The government was increasingly being pressured to do something, anything. Then corporations saw an opportunity to profit from this desperation. The history of AZT reveals the contentious relationships activists had with the pharmaceutical companies, the insurance industry, and regulatory agencies like the FDA. The worldwide sales of AZT jumped from $159 million in 1988 to over $200 million the following year. Burroughs Wellcome, AZT's manufacturer, was projected to gross $880 million from this drug by 1992. Activists in ACT UP, which was founded in New York the same month as the approval of AZT, spent their early years clamoring not only for Burroughs Wellcome to make AZT more affordable, but also for the broader drug industry and federal government to invest in other treatment options.[3]

Race and gender were also factors. AZT and later drugs were usually clinically tested on White men. Their effects on men of color and especially women were unknown. In the early 1990s, J Craig Fong was part of the AIDS Clinical Trials Group (ACTG) at the National Institute of Allergy and Infectious Diseases. "We were trying to get access to the experimental drugs to people of color," J said. "Frankly, we were fighting with a lot of the mainstream groups [on the ACTG] who were shouting, 'Me, me, me. Oh, the newest drug? I want that.'" J said these fights to get people of color onto drug trials were where he learned the vocabulary of AIDS activism, the language of racial disparity.[4]

For many AIDS activists, their vision was not just about finding a cure (or even treatment), which would be meaningless if many people couldn't afford it, but also about building a more equitable health delivery system where someone's economic status, race, or gender shouldn't determine if they could live, a precursor to universal health care.

The early history of AIDS drugs also sheds light on the anguish a person with AIDS experienced when faced with having to make life-or-death decisions about treatments, when the options were limited, when supposed experts had little advice to give, and when that advice was hard to trust. It was not uncommon for AIDS activists to become research junkies; chasing the latest peer-reviewed articles in medical journals on experimental drugs, they often became more knowledgeable than most physicians treating AIDS patients. Many ACT UP chapters had a "treatment and data committee" where members could sort out the many journal articles that were coming out about the latest discoveries. People got excited about one therapy or another that had shown some promising results with someone somewhere, but the hopes for these "cures du jour," as Napoleon Lustre dubbed them, were eventually dashed. Out of desperation, some people resorted to black-market drugs (unused supplies of AZT from those who had died, experimental drugs, hormones, etc.). The

2013 Oscar-winning film *The Dallas Buyers Club* was based on a true story about an underground smuggling network of untested AIDS drugs organized by Ron Woodruff, a person with AIDS himself. One of the therapies Woodruff pushed was Compound Q, a pure protein derived from the root of a plant in the Chinese cucumber family used to treat tumors and induce abortions. Napoleon spent a small fortune on this treatment. The FDA had not approved Compound Q because it was linked to two deaths during human trials; it was so toxic that other buyer's clubs except Woodruff's stopped dispensing it.

In the early 1990s, interleukin-2 was still an experimental drug showing some promise of increasing T-cell counts for people with HIV. Gil said that when he was working for an AIDS service organization in Honolulu, he "always knew of the people who [were] taking [interleukin-2] because their sweat would wreak of this chemical. You couldn't get it through public health. Only those that had the financial means could get that." Other dying AIDS patients resorted to buying a $7,000 machine that injected ozone gas, which some believed to have antiviral properties, into their rectum. If it had worked on one person for a short time, you could easily find someone jumping on it like it was the last lifeboat on the Titanic.[5]

In the midst of the scientific morass, some turned to spiritual or New Agey solutions. "There were all these alternative protocols," Joël Tan recalled, "the Louise Hays, the Marianne Williamsons, and *A Course in Miracles*." "Scribed" in 1976 by Helen Schucman (who claimed Jesus himself dictated the words to her), *A Course in Miracles* preached spiritual transformation based in Christian theology in the form of 365 lessons and a workbook. It continued to rise in popularity up through 1990s, especially after Williamson discussed the book on *The Oprah Winfrey Show* in 1992. Napoleon said that "that book was passed around and became everywhere in the HIV community." Joël summarized the spiritual approach: "Think positively out of dying. Think positively and your viral loads will decrease. People were really grasping at straws."

Early on, people living with HIV were pretty much left to their own devices. When Keith Kasai found out he was HIV positive in 1985, he was working for the CVS pharmacy, and he "stocked up on vitamins." "I just thought because it was an immune deficiency disease, the only way that I might be able to survive is by taking vitamins. So I took a lot of vitamins. My mother [who didn't know he was HIV positive] knew I had been sick not that long before [his diagnosis], so she just thought maybe I was just doing that so I wouldn't get sick. She didn't correlate it to anything else other than that." Keith's mother wasn't the only one in the dark either. He hadn't told his doctor about his HIV status, so he couldn't get any medical advice—not that in 1985 there was much sound medical advice to be doled out.

Keith did become sicker later, after he relocated to LA from Honolulu. By then, he had a doctor who knew about his status. He started on AZT, but he decided to ditch the regimen after six months. "My mouth tasted like metal," he recalled. "My hair fell out. I did it for as long as I could, but I just decided that it wasn't worth it for me to keep doing it."

Like Keith, Napoleon also "mega-dosed" on vitamins. He said, "Vitamin C is water soluble. It just washes out, but they came up with this good one where the body retained it and absorbed it. It was called Ester-C. I was taking four to five thousand milligrams of that a day, advised by my partner who was privately researching a lot of this. He was educating himself through the library and then later the internet. Then there was the really important newsletter that came out of San Francisco, *Project Inform*, which was one of the first really to keep up and break down clinical trials of the pharmaceutical companies. It would tell people how to enroll in experimental [trials]."

In the local Asian American community, some resorted to alternative and traditional medicine. Stanley Rebultan, Asian/Pacific Lesbians and Gays president in its early years, became what Napoleon called a "loud proponent" of bitter melon therapy. Gil remembered that Rebultan claimed that it had rid his system of the virus. Bitter melon (*ampalaya* in Tagalog and *kugua* in Mandarin), according to Ric, is purported to have "antiviral properties." "I know that in the Philippines, mothers give bitter melon juice to the newborn babies to kick in their immune system." He was juicing it and drinking it like a tea, and to him, it tasted even nastier than it sounded. "It was so green. It was packed full of chlorophyll."[6]

Ric went on to explain that "Stanley Rebultan's regimen was to boil it, let it cool, and then do it rectally." Like an enema. The method confused some people. Ric said some people forgot to let the solution cool the first time and ended up shooting almost-boiling water up their asses.

Joël also had a bitter melon story from an early Asian Pacific AIDS Intervention Team (APAIT) client. The client told Joël that he thought the bitter melon therapy was working but complained that "it hurts so much." When Joël asked him if he was juicing the gourd, the client looked at him and said, "You're supposed to juice it?" It turned out that he was shoving the bitter melon up his anus. Instead of an enema, the client had been using it like a dildo. "Something's working, girl," responded Joël, "but I don't think it's what you think."

Besides bitter melon, Ric also tried Chinese herbal medicine to manage his viral load:

> When we started out at APAIT, our office was right there in China-town. I just prayed to the goddesses, "Let me find somebody," and I walked right into this Chinese pharmacy [apothecary shop]. I found this doctor who would do traditional Chinese medicine and asked him if he treated people with HIV. Lo and behold, he already had a client base. The universe took me where I needed to be. I guess in China, it's about who your patients are. They'd trust you if you have prominent patients, so he immediately showed me his [HIV-positive] patient list. Confidentiality wasn't even a factor. I was shocked. I was like, "No, no, no, no, no. Don't show me that." I saw some friends on that list, and some pretty prominent people, too. He barely spoke English.

The doctor barked a few English words at him—"Sit. Tongue. Hand."— and Ric obliged. "The first time, he took a look at my tongue, he felt my pulse. That told him everything about me. Then he put together this conglomeration of leaves and all kinds of stuff and told me to boil it in a clay pot. I did it for a while."

Knowing what he knew about holistic medicine, Ric suspected that the doctor was not just treating his HIV. He said, "He would always tell me, 'No drink cold water. Only warm water.' He told me I had too much heat. Or he pointed down there [crotch area], 'no power' and then he said, 'I help you.' I don't know if it worked, but I'm here talking to you now when they had told me I had two years to live."

As he kept up with the latest research, Ric began to systematize his knowledge and share it with APAIT clients. In doing so, he slowly created a new field of direct services that came to be called "treatment advocacy." Shawn Griffin, of the Gay Men of Color Consortium, dubbed Ric "one of the parents of treatment advocacy," and APAIT had named its treatment library after Ric. Ric credited the PLUS (Positive Living for Us) weekend seminar, established in the mid-1980s by Shanti, another AIDS service organization, for giving him the inspiration for the idea. He had participated in the seminar at the urging of Joël shortly after they met. "Basically, it was a boot camp for people with HIV," he said. "It was a series of workshops and lectures. Starting with medical updates, alternative therapies, insurance and public benefits, meditation. All kinds of things that you would need to know. Over three days. It raised my awareness that I have the right to know what's going on with my body, a right to make informed decisions. It was really about consciousness raising, and changing this dynamic of helplessness."

Because all the funding streams had to be tied to an established service category determined by the AIDS commission, APAIT was initially unable to get funding from the county for this line of work. But the agency didn't give up. People living with HIV had so many questions, some that they didn't even know how to ask. The need was simply immense.

It was only going to get more complicated until the scientific community found out more about the disease. By the early 1990s, the mainstream medical community admitted that AZT alone wasn't effective for most patients but that it could have some benefits when combined with other drugs. What complicated matters was that everybody reacted differently to the symptoms of AIDS, partly because AIDS is not technically a disease but rather a syndrome involving a severely weakened immune system, which makes people with HIV more susceptible to diseases that other humans never have to worry about. People don't die from AIDS. They die from complications of AIDS, from "opportunistic infections," the most common of which are Kaposi's sarcoma (a type of cancer) and pneumocystis pneumonia (PCP). People who were taking drugs to control their viral loads were often taking other kinds of medications to treat these complications.

In 1988, after AZT went on the market, the FDA approved trimetrexate to treat PCP, alpha interferon for Kaposi's sarcoma, and ganciclovir for cytomegalovirus retinitis. In 1989 came aerosolized pentamidine for PCP, another drug for cytomegalovirus retinitis, erythropoietin to treat anemia as a result of AZT, and dideoxyinosine (ddI) for AIDS patients who were intolerant of AZT. In 1990, Diflucan (fluconazole) to treat AIDS-related fungal infections, and another drug for AZT-related anemia appeared. And these were just a few drugs that the most conscientious physicians (and just as often, vigilant activists) had to keep abreast of.

The interactions from multiple drugs might create a kaleidoscope of side effects on different bodies, none of which could be known until someone tried the combination and saw what would manifest. Finding a right combination was pretty much a private trial-and-error hell, where most people had to experience nausea, fatigue, hair loss, or diarrhea in order to figure out that something was not working and that they should move on to a different combination, experimenting until they settled not on the perfect combo, but on a lesser evil. Your health condition has changed? Your combination would also have to change. And the side effects did not dissipate over time; if anything, the virus often became resistant to the drugs, losing effectiveness but not the effects. The side effects could be so severe that some patients decided not to comply. If they were going to die sooner or later, they reasoned, they could at least spend their last months with some quality of life and dignity.

Even when a patient was motivated for full adherence to a perfectly customized protocol, they were confronted with a set of instructions on how to take these drugs that would be complicated even for someone with sound health and mind. And that person was tethered to the drug-taking schedule. In the early 1990s, when his T-cells started to dip below five hundred, Gil decided to enroll in one of the earliest clinical trials for protease inhibitors (the drug that would soon make AIDS a manageable disease). "My fucking God, that was horrible," he recalled. "It was eight pills, three times a day"—relatively straightforward in those days—"taken with water. It gave me fatigue and dizziness and diarrhea. There was never any education on how to take the pills. No advice." Just when Gil got the hang of the regimen, he and his partner, Juan, decided to move forward with their plan to go hiking in Yosemite. "I didn't have enough water," said Gil. "The medication got stuck in my throat all the time. I was gagging from this stuff. Plus, I was fatigued. I was dragging this backpack and nearly slipping off these trails at the same time." These live-and-learn moments were common as people struggled to balance making life adjustments and retaining some semblance of normalcy.

Treatment advocates tried to minimize this anguish by helping AIDS patients wade through the muddy water of treatment options and make the most informed decision. Ric explained, "We needed to help people figure out what were the real treatments and what were the bogus quackery. People were getting taken advantage of because they were so scared." Then there was a more holistic wellness approach: yoga, meditation, traditional Chinese medicine; "All of those started to gain popularity." Ric had his opinions based on his own experience, but as a treatment advocate, he tried to remain objective and give the clients the information they needed to arrive at their own conclusions. After all, the goal was to help clients feel more in charge of their treatment. "We never ever tell people what they should or should not be doing," he explained. "We said, 'This is what we know. Right? This is what we don't know. These are the possible side effects. This is the history of that drug company, how they've behaved in the community. These are the alternatives. This is what your insurance will pay for.' It demystified the whole realm [of AIDS treatment] so people weren't afraid of it anymore."

Under Ric's guidance in the mid-1990s, Gil went from being a client at APAIT to being a treatment advocate. "I never told anyone not to [try a medication] because I wanted them to hold onto hope," Gil said. "If someone felt that this or that particular herb was helping them, it could be the placebo effect. Maybe that's all it takes. The mental process, I believe, helps someone go through other challenges of surviving the disease, the will to say, 'I'm not going to be defeated.'"

A top complaint of any health-care consumer has always been not having enough time with their doctor, who is probably burdened not only by the number of patients they have to see every hour, but also by the paperwork required to document each visit. When people with AIDS finally got their face time with a doctor, shame might deter some from asking too many questions. For many immigrants, the language barrier complicated the client-caregiver interaction even more. Treatment advocates sometimes escorted their clients to their medical appointments, according to Gil, "because they're not going to understand what their doctor says. They got fifteen minutes with the doctor, maybe twenty if they're lucky. Then afterwards, they'd say, 'Okay, that was a blur. What did the doctor actually say?'" As a treatment advocate, Gil would break it down and develop a plan with them.

"No one was teaching them how to develop a plan for taking their medications," Gil said. "Well, you'd hear a doctor say, 'Take these three pills five times a day. Take this one three times a day, but you have to have food. Now this one over here, you have to do it two times a day without food.' There is no conceptual sense from the medical provider of what that meant on a day-to-day process." To help the clients, Gil would draw a clock (two concentric circle, one representing AM, and the other PM) on a piece of paper and indicate which pills (color-coded) to take at what time.

Shawn Griffin also saw treatment advocacy as a way to address class disparity in access to quality care:

> The less money a client had, the less time they were able to spend with their doctor. They'd come in and see the doctor, the doctor would look at them, shake their heads a couple times, and say take this twice a day. If there were side effects, if they couldn't get up in the morning because the medication made them so tired, so groggy, if they couldn't keep the food down, the doctor kept telling them there was nothing they could do, that they just had to take it and suffer through. They really lived in the dark. The whole idea behind treatment advocacy was to really give the client a role in their own treatment, so they didn't feel like a bystander. Sometimes the treatment advocate would even help them come up with questions they could ask their doctor, to get more information.

Treatment advocates also encouraged clients not to accept any pat responses from their doctors. By empowering AIDS patients, treatment advocacy challenged the unquestioned authority of the medical community. The medical community was not used to patients asking too many questions, and many physicians had a "just-do-what-I-say" attitude. This was especially poignant for women living with HIV. Because women often have different AIDS symptoms and most of the research and clinic experiences focused on men, providers could miss how fast the disease was progressing in their female patients. Staff remember an early APAIT client, a Chinese American woman, who died "suddenly" because her doctor had not taken her complaints seriously. Ric said, "The arrogance was breathtaking when you were dealing with a lot of these doctors and clinicians."

Because both Ric and Gil were HIV positive, their experience with the virus was an asset for treatment advocacy, but it didn't shield them from the mental strain. Gil explained, "I knew that I was observing something that I might experience in the future. I would always stop myself from projecting, 'This could be me!' At the forefront in my service delivery was compassion, that I can do as much as I can to help this individual have the best quality of life that they could possibly experience. It was hard and often traumatic." Yet when Gil came out of retirement in 2006, he came back "with the caveat that I only wanted to do hands-on work, I only wanted to be a treatment advocate."

APAIT couldn't keep supporting treatment advocacy out of its discretionary fund, not at the scale that it was needed. They knew they had to get the AIDS commission to recognize treatment advocacy as a necessary service. But at that point, Ric recalled, money was tight, and "people were like, 'No, you're wasting money on that [treatment advocacy]. We need money for this or that.'" Weren't doctors giving patients all the information they needed? Weren't case managers already coordinating all their services? Ric continued:

> People didn't know what it was, so we gave them street theater. We showed up [at the AIDS commission] and I had written this thing, kind of like a poem, basically all the questions that patients would ask us. What is AZT? What is this? What is that? Why should I talk to my doctor? I can't talk to my doctor because I don't trust him. It was all bullet points of conversations that I had had with clients.
>
> There were probably 150 people in the room, and about 40 people at the council table. I just kept reading and reading and reading. At the end, the whole room was dead silent. Then this Dr. [Wilbert] Jordan— he was the most vocal opponent of treatment advocacy—was the first to speak. "There's no secret that I've been against treatment advocacy. But after hearing from that young man, I'm happy to announce that

I'm fully 100 percent in favor of treatment advocacy." The whole room just lit up. That was the turning point, when the county actually made a proclamation that they would fund it as a service category.

Slowly, others in the AIDS service spectrum began to see the benefits of treatment advocacy. "What we noticed," Ric explained, "was that when the knowledge goes up, [medication] adherence goes up. They were no longer afraid of it." When people started to take their medications correctly—especially as the medications were progressively getting better—their health improved. Gil remembered getting feedback from a social worker at the Gay and Lesbian Community Services Center with whom he shared some clients in common. The social worker said, "Boy, without your services, we would be swamped, because the doctors get fifteen minutes before the next patient came in. So they referred their patients to me to do the follow-up education on medication." Even some doctors came around. Some started coming to the seminars Ric organized, saying, "Yeah, I want to participate in this because I'm having better conversations with my patients."

In 1995, Ric and Gil took the show on the road. Their proposal to present on treatment advocacy at the US Conference on AIDS was accepted. It was the largest gathering of scientists, activists, physicians, and policymakers working on AIDS, drawing thousands for skill building, networking, and information sharing. Perhaps because the organizers thought the topic wouldn't attract a lot of conference participants, Ric and Gil's workshop was assigned to the more remote part of the venue. Gil recalled that "they put us in this warehouse area. The chairs all looked different. Ric and I were saying, 'God, how are people going to find us?' We had a hard time finding that place."

Nevertheless, people started showing up, and gradually, the room filled to capacity. "It was standing room only," Gil said, as he and Ric found themselves facing the opposite problem. "Right in front of us was the LA County director of health services, who was also responsible for overseeing the Commission on HIV and AIDS. She was staring right at us, and I said to Ric, under my breath, 'Oh, my fucking God.' Talk about being nervous!"

Ric remembered that they had only come up with an activity that very morning. As people were filing in, they had given them each a packet of candies in different colors, along with a small sheet of instructions. The participants were directed to eat a certain color of candies at different intervals throughout the session. At this point in our interview, Gil stood up and filed back and forth the ten feet in his living room, holding an imaginary microphone. "First we got into a spiel about the basics, about how the advances of medication had brought us to the point of having multiple options. Then we were walking up and down the aisle and asking people to share their experience [working with people with AIDS]. At the end of the presentation, I said, 'Oh, by the way, ladies and gentlemen. Recall the little packets I gave you with the instruction? Those are the medications you dispense to your patients. How many of you remembered to follow those instructions?'" The audience were so focused on the presentation that most had forgotten that part of the workshop. "Immediately, you would see their faces. They got it," Gil said. "They understood the difficulty, the importance of developing some protocol so the patients would adhere once they leave the medical office."

Even Big Pharma wanted a piece of it eventually. They started to offer funding to agencies like APAIT to gather their clients to learn about the latest advances in *their* AIDS medication. They would even cater these workshops, a drop in the large bucket that was their marketing budget. Gil offered this reflection: "I don't think it's ever going to be a situation where there's compassionate development of medication. There's always a profit motive behind it. It was convenient for pharmaceuticals to jump on the bandwagon. They profited quite a bit and continued to do so."

Diep Tran, who joined APAIT in the mid-1990s, offered the example of Marinol (dronabinol), a synthetic drug with a similar compound to marijuana that is used to treat debilitating AIDS symptoms. A typical prescription of sixty 2.5-milligram capsules costs about $250. "It was to help you with your pain and also be able to increase your appetite," said Diep. "It's pretty much just marijuana. Why the fuck do you need it in pill form? A lot of us queers were like, 'Fuck these pharmaceuticals. Why not just legalize marijuana?' It irked me that people had to pay for something that in theory they could have grown themselves. And even the ads about Marinol, where the fuck is the queer in this?"

Joël added, "Big Pharma, capitalism in general, was the enemy. . . . There was a patriarchy that was fucking with us, and it needed to be shut down. They obstructed the trajectory of cure. The whole idea about cure research was overwhelmed by the pharmaceutical enterprise." Even in 2018, BioSpace.com, a digital hub for news, insights, and opportunities for the life sciences industry, wrote about the state of "the growing HIV market." The article concluded, "While companies are all vying for a slice of the HIV market share, Gilead, which earned $14 billion from its HIV pipeline last year, could be on its way to actually finally an effective cure for the disease. . . . Any potential human trial results are years away though and the company's HIV pipeline is safe for the time being."[7] Considering how much profit these companies were generating from people with HIV managing their chronic condition, the statement seemed like they were more urgently interested in the safety of a dominant HIV pipeline than in finding a cure.

At the same time, Gil acknowledged, the treatment research done by these companies did begin to yield better drugs in the mid-1990s that offered many people living with HIV—Gil, included—not only longevity, but also a better quality of life. By 1996, the scientists had figured out that a cocktail of medications that included antiretrovirals (which is what AZT was), non-nucleoside reverse transcriptase inhibitors, and protease inhibitors (the latest innovation at the time) could help stabilize a patient's T-cell counts with far fewer side effects. As uneasy as the relationship with Big Pharma was, there was no way not to have a relationship with it. As Gil concluded, "There's nothing you can do about that."

Sure enough, the activists began to notice the increasing presence of the pharmaceutical companies in the 1990s. Not only were they sponsoring conferences and plastering their brands all over, but also, as Joël said, "they stopped just going for the doctors and started to work on case managers. All of a sudden, Glaxo Wellcome [formed in 1995 by a merger between AZT manufacturer Burroghs Wellcome and Glaxo] was taking you out to dinners, in the same way they do with doctors. You would be wined and dined so that you can recommend their drugs. Those motherfuckers are really something."

Ric also observed that "the pharmaceutical companies started fighting back by throwing money at it. Suddenly, these treatment advocates were being flown all over the country to different conferences. 'Oh, we want you to educate your population, and here's a ticket to Miami, and here's the hotel.'" Pharmaceutical companies had always courted physicians to promote their drugs with their patients—this is why we have an opioid epidemic now—and the fact that they were targeting case managers and treatment advocates illustrates the growing influence of people in these positions on those living with HIV.

Initially, Ric was able to secure some funding from Big Pharma without falling into the traps of pushing their products. Nevertheless, the infiltration of drug money defanged the potency of treatment advocacy. Ric noticed that people who bought into the approach started to call themselves treatment "educators" rather than the more assertive "advocates." In other words, clients needed to be educated about what was good for them, not empowered to ask questions. Ric said, "The doctors still didn't like the idea of patient empowerment. When they switched it to treatment education because they didn't like the word advocacy, it lost its power. After that, it just kind of dissipated."

By shifting the focus to managing AIDS as a chronic condition, advances in AIDS medicines in the mid-1990s further contributed to the waning of the movement. None of the activists begrudges the companies for developing more effective drugs that helped people with HIV live longer and attain a better quality of life. Yet they bemoan the loss of a radical critique of our health delivery system from the early AIDS movement.

CHAPTER 12

That Shrinking Window of Reconciliation

IN THE EARLY 1980S, KEITH KASAI HAD A GIRLFRIEND. THEY WERE both in their twenties. She wasn't his first, but a series of heterosexual relationships, dating back to his high school days, didn't stop him from cruising public parks in Hawai'i, looking for sex with other men. The rumor of a disease affecting gay men was beginning to drift across the Pacific, and the small cluster of locals with whom Keith hung around in the park whispered it among themselves. The guys, ethnic Chinese and Japanese who grew up on Oahu, dismissed it as a mainland scourge. "Just don't have sex with *haoles* or tourists," they advised one another and went on with their business as usual.

The brush-off did not sit well with Keith. Tourists have sex with locals, a fact as old and irrefutable as tourism itself. He knew local people could contract the virus, but he didn't air his concerns. He, too, went on with his business as usual.

When the HIV antibody test became available in Hawai'i in 1985, the group made a pact to go get tested at the Diamond Head Health Center. Back then, it took a week to get the result, and many people, fearful of bad news, would not go back to find out their status. To make each other accountable, Keith's friends decided to meet one night to share their results. Keith had to work late that night. By the time he reached the group, everyone had disclosed their status. All of them were negative.

Except for Keith.

Keith kept his positive status to himself. "Oahu is a small island," he explained. "I was afraid of people talking. I didn't want to be the center of the gossip."

He didn't even consult a doctor. The only person he told was his girlfriend, who had known about his dalliances with men. Neither quite grasped the severity of the situation, and they continued to have unprotected sex. Blame it on the lack of public HIV education or their young libido. Thankfully, she never became positive.

In 1986, Keith and his girlfriend moved to LA. Their cohabitation wasn't working from the beginning. The uncertainty of his prognosis hung over him and sped up his coming out. Before they broke up, his younger brother followed him to LA and stayed with them. One night, Keith told his brother that he was splitting up with his girlfriend, that he was not only gay but also HIV positive. Although Keith had made it clear that he wasn't ready to tell their parents, and that even when that time came, it would be him who would do the telling, his brother thought their parents had a right to know. And the three-hour time difference just made the hour decent enough to call home after Keith went to bed that night.

The next night when he came home from work, Keith still had no clue that his brother had outed him, but the awkward silence between his girlfriend and his brother tipped him off that something was wrong. The phone rang and broke the silence. Once he picked up the phone, his father's yelling made him wish for the silence to return.

"He was pissed that I'm gay," Keith recalled. "He couldn't even say the word *gay*. He just said, 'I can't believe you moved out there to be like that.'" Though Keith did not hear from his mother that night, his father let him know in no uncertain terms that she was upset. So upset, in fact, that her vocal cords tightened up and she couldn't even talk to him.

His father continued the tirade: "How could you do this to us? What am I going to tell my friends? I would rather you had called me from jail and told me you need money to get bailed out than to hear you're like that."

Keith would hear from his mother five months later, in a letter. She was not as belligerent as his father; she was more worried that Keith would lose his job or be killed. Nevertheless, her disapproval dismayed Keith so much that he threw the letter away.

In our interview three decades later at his home in Studio City, I asked Keith if either of his parents had any worries about his HIV status back in 1987.

"No," he answered. "The main focus was me being gay and what they're going to tell people." He followed this with a story about his father's cousin, whom the locals would consider a *mahu*. His family did not know until "he had gone to the bars and came back home in drag." The brothers beat him up; the mother took him to a psychiatrist to fix him. Keith shared this story, as if to explain how the brutal reactions to his relative's sexuality had become a prototype for his parents.

Much later, after Keith and his parents were talking again, he found out during one of his visits home that his father had "punched holes in the walls" after he discovered that Keith was gay. When he looked behind new picture frames on these walls, he found evidence of this rage. Keith was glad that they had been an ocean apart. "It wouldn't surprise me that my dad would have beaten me," he said. Keith had known that his dad, as a child, was abused by his father, even if his dad wouldn't recognize it as such. Keith said, "There's one story my dad tells me. When my dad and uncle were little, they would chase each other around the yard. One time, my dad jumped into the car, rolled up the windows and locked the doors. My uncle hit the window and cracked it. My grandfather tied them both up to the mango tree and hit them with a belt. That's old school. My dad reminded me how lucky we were that we weren't tied to the tree. But he still hit us, anyway. These things just stick with you. There were good times, but there were some pretty shitty times. This is one of the reasons why I wanted to get out of the house."

By the time Keith's parents learned about his HIV status in 1987, the AIDS hysteria had not been quelled. AZT, AIDS's first fast-tracked drug, had barely been approved, and the public image of a person with AIDS was an emaciated man with blotches of lesions. Keith was given a prognosis of five years when he was diagnosed in 1985. Their fixation on Keith's sexual orientation at the expense of his HIV status—and his health—seemed misplaced to me. AIDS was an imminent death sentence to many in those years, but it was unemployment or a hate crime that his mother feared would cut his life short?

This was how deep homophobia cut. As much as public health officials and some AIDS activists tried to dissociate gayness from AIDS, a lot of AIDS activism was about confronting homophobia. In those years, when they could not save many from a certain death, AIDS workers made sure that people at least did not die alone or with regrets, but with dignity and support.

After the break-up, Keith remained in LA without much of a support network. With the prognosis clock ticking, he admitted to being "a little careless" with his life: drinking, doing drugs, racking up credit card debts. He thought, "I'm going to be dead. So what's the point?"

Then in 1989 he met a man named Eric, in the steam room at the Sports Connection, a cruisy gym in West Hollywood. They dated for a while. Though the relationship didn't last, they've remained friends to this day. Eric had been involved in ACT UP/LA, and Keith began to participate in direct actions with him.

"They were trying to get better health care for people with AIDS. I felt, as a person with HIV, that I wanted to be there with them. Whenever they needed people to hold signs, I was there. I remember carrying the 'Silence = Death' sign, in West Hollywood and downtown. We had stopped traffic at the intersections."

Through ACT UP/LA, Keith connected with Shanti, an organization that provided emotional support to people with HIV. At first, he wasn't comfortable going to a support group to talk about his feelings. Instead, he trained to be a group facilitator. Facilitation freed him from the expectation to disclose, and it gave him a window into how other people were coping with the virus, while helping others in the process.

The irony of someone not emotionally ready to talk about his plight leading a group of people in a discussion about the very same plight felt familiar to me. Many Asian Americans, Keith thought, are made reticent by their cultural upbringing to disclose personal stories to a group of strangers. But when given a defined role, they may find themselves open to things that are too scary to explore otherwise.

Even though Keith had lived with HIV for almost five years by then, the facilitation experience opened his eyes to the disease:

Everybody was in a different stage of HIV. It was hard for me as well as for people who had just gotten tested to see people walk in with full-blown AIDS or KS spots all over. People kept leaving because they were getting sicker. Or they would never come back. I'd call and then I'd find out that they had passed. As a facilitator, I was the one who had to keep passing on this news that so-and-so's gone or so-and-so's really sick. It was just this constant flux of people. Sometimes we never got a chance to say goodbye.

For the first time, Keith got to see, firsthand, how fast the disease moved. Keith realized that "it's okay to be afraid, it's okay to need someone to talk to, because it's not good to hold everything in."

Shanti was also where Keith met his partner, Peter.

In his early AIDS activism, Keith hardly ever found another Asian American in a support group or at a direct action. So he deliberately took on more visible roles. One year, he went on the ACT UP/LA float in the gay pride parade. He recalled, "I was on this huge float by myself in a blue dress with white stars and a tiara, waving to people as the song 'Don't Leave Me This Way' played on a loop. It was pretty funny."

One night in the early 1990s, Keith ran into a friend from Hawai'i, and through him, Keith met Tracy Nako, another transplant from the Aloha State. Tracy and Keith instantly bonded over being "local boys" in LA. Tracy had also just started working at Asian Pacific AIDS Intervention Team (APAIT). By that time, Keith had no qualms about revealing his status. It wasn't long before Tracy recruited him to be a volunteer.

Most volunteers at the time helped out with street outreach and passing out condoms to patrons at gay bars and clubs. Because of his HIV status, Keith was asked to do more. When APAIT rolled out its "Love Your Asian Body" campaign (1992) to promote HIV testing, Keith agreed to be a model. In postcards and advertisements, he was shown in an erotic straddle with Eric Reyes, another APAIT volunteer. Both were naked. Although their private parts were artfully hidden, their joyful faces were clearly visible in these images.

Keith's own motivation to be one of the very public Asian faces of HIV wasn't that different from what got him onto a gay pride float. "At that time, there was nobody that wanted to be out, as far as being HIV and Asian. People don't want to be correlated with being gay or having AIDS, having your face on the [post]cards." Before his AIDS activism, he was living recklessly with what he thought was his limited time on earth. While his expiration date was no less uncertain, Keith now lived with a purpose. He said, "I didn't know how long I was going to live. I might as well be useful."

When APAIT found a gay Asian man who was willing to talk about being HIV positive, they glommed onto him. On behalf of the agency, Keith was profiled in *Rafu Shimpo* to raise AIDS awareness in the Asian American community. He was dispatched as a speaker on a panel—almost always the only Asian American, and often the only person of color—to share his experience. As he stayed healthy after the first five years, Keith moved the goalpost to ten. He kept volunteering, taking one assignment after the next. "Once I started volunteering, I became more and more comfortable doing it," he said. He also thought that being so far away from the rest of his family in Hawai'i offered him a shield of anonymity that others in LA couldn't wield.

Keith soon discovered just how connected the communities in Hawai'i and LA were, even with the Pacific Ocean between them. Keith was featured in APAIT's next social marketing campaign, "Facing HIV and AIDS." For this, Keith appeared, fully clothed this time, with a group of Asian Americans, including both men and women, from diverse ethnic groups and across the age spectrum. The picture was captioned by the statement, "Two of Them Have HIV." Keith was one of them, but you could never tell from the wholesome lineup. Appearing "normal" and "healthy," the models together tried to debunk the myth that HIV could be contracted only by a certain demographic group or that you could tell if someone was HIV positive solely by looking at them.

Keith said, "My brother's friend saw the billboard, recognized me, called my brother. And of course, my brother called my mother and said, 'Keith's on a billboard.' My mother called me and said, 'Why do you have to do these things?'"

To this, Keith shared a refrain that had become familiar: "Because nobody else would do it."

Having a community—a "chosen family," as many LGBTQ people call our non-biological support network—kept Keith healthy in the early

1990s. The APAIT family really came through once Keith fell ill in 1993, after he had just moved in with Peter. Keith recounted that time:

> I was home sick and Tracy checked up on me. I had a fever of 102. He came over, picked me up, and took me to the doctor. Then I found out I had spinal meningitis and shingles. It was lucky I had gone to the hospital, because they did the T-cell count on me. My T-cell count was 60. They gave me an AIDS diagnosis, because it was under 100. Afterwards, while recuperating at home, they [APAIT] had their in-house therapist, Margaret Endo, come to my house and visit me. She came over like four times in six weeks. I thought this was the beginning of the end, so pretty much what we talked about was, "How do you deal with this?"

Keith the APAIT volunteer became Keith the APAIT client. After years of activism, Keith finally could share his fears and anxieties with someone.

Margaret Endo Shimada was APAIT's first clinical staff member, once the agency finally received funding for mental health counseling. By the time she joined APAIT, Margaret was an experienced clinician, having worked at the Asian American Drug Abuse Program (AADAP) and Keiro, a community-based organization that served Japanese American older adults. However, she was a novice when it came to AIDS. Her one introduction to the disease had come ten years before, when Sally Jue fought her way to make a presentation to AADAP staff in the early 1980s, warning them that they were about to confront one of the most devastating epidemics in their lifetimes. Since then, Margaret had not had to deal with people with AIDS either personally or professionally. She was a little perplexed when she received a call from Naomi Kageyama.

"[Naomi] said they were looking for a clinical person for this project," Margaret recalled. "She said, 'You might be a good fit.' But I knew nothing about the gay and lesbian community. And what I had learned was such a small snippet of what this whole crisis was about." Margaret nevertheless consented to meeting both Naomi and Dean. At the interview, she reiterated her lack of experience, telling Dean, "I don't know how I can help you guys." To this, Dean replied, "We just need a clinical person that can help us talk to people."

There was a limited pool of people with both the clinical experience and the experience working with people with AIDS or the LGBTQ Asian American community in general. The mental health field had not been friendly to queer people, and the wind had only begun to shift in the 1970s. Clinicians like Terry Gock and Sally Jue who had been doing AIDS advocacy for over a decade by the early 1990s were truly exceptional, and these folks were also far enough along in their career path that they were unavailable for a starting position at APAIT. Many in the new generation of Asian American AIDS activists had not considered this as their career choice, though some would eventually go back to graduate school in social work or public health as the AIDS field became more professionalized. In the meantime, APAIT had to look outside of their network to build out their clinical practice.

The position was part time. Pregnant with her first child, Margaret thought she had time for this challenge. She explained, "It's the same reason I took on the job at AADAP and Keiro. I had gone into social work to help people, to serve the community. That's what I enjoy doing. I went in not thinking I could really make an impact, but I was going to learn and grow from this experience, and then hopefully make an impact at some point."

In our interview, Margaret described her motive as "self-serving," but "I'm here to learn" was the perfectly humble approach to reach this stigmatized population. She said, "I didn't go in thinking, 'I'm the expert, and I'm going to show everybody, teach everybody.' I've always felt in social work, maybe in life, you have to start at the ground level and really be able to work through and understand what the issues are."

Her first task was to formalize the counseling services. For this she turned to Yoshi Matsuhima for help. A pioneer licensed clinical social worker in the Asian American community, Matsuhima had managed the Coastal Asian Pacific Mental Health Services program at the LA County Department of Mental Health. Margaret and he met every other week to figure out how to "format the counseling services." Their collaboration convinced her to keep and formalize the support groups that Ric and Sally started, while developing a new individual counseling program. Margaret also recognized that she needed to complement Matsuhima's technical expertise with real-life experiences. She counted on Ric as "a big resource." She said, "Ric was just Ric. I was really green. He was always extending himself. "

Others at the agency became part of her education, too. Because they shared many clients in common, Margaret worked closely with Tracy Nako, the case manager. They often made home visits to clients together. "I remember driving to a home visit with Tracy in my car. It was pouring rain, and my heater went out, and we were both freezing. I had these blankets in the car that we piled on ourselves. I was pregnant. It was a mess, but it's what you do. We were in it together."

She had wanted to do a couples' therapy group, but she was fretting how to approach gay relationships since she had never worked with gay couples before. Dean told her, "As couples, we have the same issues as anyone else." That helped take some of the pressure off Margaret. She said, "Talking to Ric, talking to Tracy, talking with Dean, that's the only way to learn."

Margaret had counseled enough people with serious illnesses to know their challenges in communication, grieving, guilt, and anger. "People were just looking for a place where they can just talk and share," she said. "And maybe the fact that I was outside the community, that made it easier." Sure enough, Margaret found that in the couples' support group, people were dealing with familiar issues of trust and communication. "And chores," she added. "Who's doing the chores and who isn't?"

But the "prick-us-and-we-also-bleed" approach had its limits. We are the same as everyone else, until we are not. One-on-one, learning more in-depth the lives of people with AIDS, was where Margaret encountered her biggest learning curve. One of her favorite clients was this "really charming and engaging" sansei (third-generation Japanese American). Margaret said, "He told me he went to these support groups called SCA. I said, 'SCA, what is that?' He said, 'Sexually Compulsives Anonymous.' I had no idea. He had a number of partners, while he was HIV positive, but he was in a committed relationship. What did that mean for his partner? What did that mean for these other men that he was having these relationships with? He and his partner came together a couple of times for therapy. His partner was asking, 'You're having sex with all these different people. How do you think that makes me feel?'"

Whatever she needed to learn, she needed to do it quickly. When her clients started going downhill, the progression was swift. When Margaret had to make home visits for those who couldn't come to her, she knew it was time to help the clients be at peace with the inevitable end. That was how she had met Keith, at his home.

But luckily, it turned out to be a false alarm for Keith. After more than a month of those dark expectations at home, he started to get better.

As Keith was nursed back to health, he began to think about reconciliation with his parents. Perhaps it was the bout with mortality that had pushed him to think about this. By then, there was some communication, and definitely willingness on the other side. "They would come and visit me," Keith explained, "but I wouldn't want to go home [to Hawaiʻi]. It was always awkward, because I was dating women in Hawaiʻi. They were curious as to why I moved to LA, and all of a sudden, this [being gay]. They'd ask, 'How do you know?' I knew because I had three girlfriends and I had sex with all three of them. I knew who I was, and it wasn't going to change."

Keith's parents continued to "barrage [him] with 'Have you met a nice girl? We'll fix you up.'" Keith said, "I told my parents, 'I'm going to tell everybody because I'm tired of lying to Grandma and Grandpa. They were like, 'Don't you dare!' I did, anyway. And nobody cared. The only people that cared was my parents because they were worried about what people were going to say about them. My grandparents didn't care. They just said, 'Oh, okay.' Maybe they said something to my parents, but they never said anything to me. But at least now [my parents] stopped asking me about dating girls."

With a solid relationship with Peter, Keith decided to visit his parents with his boyfriend. In private, his parents had "warmed up to [Peter] because he was just a really nice guy, open and with a sense of humor." In public, things had not changed much. Once, Keith introduced Peter as his partner to his parents' neighbor. The next day, Keith and his mother had the following exchange:

MRS. KASAI: Why did you tell her you were gay?
KEITH: I didn't tell her I was gay. I just introduced Peter as my partner.
MRS. KASAI: Well, you can be gay. Just don't tell people.

KEITH: What do you want me to say, Mom? Do you want me to say, "This is Peter, the gardener? This is Peter, the garbage man? This is Peter, my roommate?"

For Keith, the kicker was when his mother called him a couple of years later to tell him that her neighbor, the one that Keith had supposedly come out to, had been cheating on her husband and had separated from him as a result. He was mad that his mother was doing the exact kind of gossiping that she was afraid others would do about her family. "I told her, 'You were so worried about what this woman next door was going to think of you, when here she is, fooling around behind her husband's back and their three little kids.' Really? This is who you find more important?'"

Homophobia cuts deep, but it also spreads wide. When many of us who are LGBTQ come out to our parents, we suddenly let go of some of the shame and paranoia, and immediately we see them latching onto our parents. They're the ones who now incubate it. They're the ones who are afraid of other people finding out. In some ways, homophobia is very much like a virus.

And like HIV, homophobia writhes when exposed to open air.

Once, when his parents were in LA, Keith received an invitation from Dean Goishi to bring them to a meeting at the residence of Ellen and Harold Kameya. In the 1990s, the Kameyas were already something of a legend in the LGBTQ Asian American community in LA. Their daughter Valerie had come out to them in the late 1980s. They had reacted with sadness and disappointment. "Valerie's announcement devastated us," wrote Harold Kameya in 2010. "At that time, we were woefully ignorant on issues of sexual orientation, including that being gay is not a choice. As part of that ignorance, we were saddened that we would never see our daughter get married or have a family."

Feeling isolated, the Kameyas sought out their local P-FLAG (Parents and Friends of Lesbians and Gays) chapter. They were the only Asian Americans at these meetings. In 1990, they shared their story of transformation with an eager group of young LGBTQ Asian Americans. Harold wrote of this "turning point": "After we spoke, we were moved by the tears on the faces of the audience. They told us of the pain that gays and lesbians faced."[1] Afterward, the Kameyas "felt compelled to break the silence in our community." In public, they took on more speaking engagements. In private, they held spaces for LGBTQ Asian Americans and their parents. The Kameyas fashioned a proto-P-FLAG at their home so that other Asian American parents wouldn't have to experience the isolation they had felt. Back then, many of us would gladly take private acceptance from our parents; any public acknowledgment would be a pipe dream. In that way, Keith's parents were the norms. From the Kameyas, we learned that we deserved more and not to take only scraps.

Keith knew that his parents wouldn't go to the meeting at the Kameyas' if he had asked them directly. His parents had other opportunities to reach out for support. As it turned out, besides the *mahu* uncle, Keith had a lesbian cousin. Keith said, "But yet, her father and my father would not talk about what's happening. You would think they'd want somebody to talk to. But, no. So they're not going to go [to the Kameyas']. I know them."

Instead, Keith asked them to come with him to run an errand, a request just vague enough for them to accept. The trick worked, to a point.

"When we pulled into the [Kameyas'] house, my dad asked, 'Why are we here?' Of course, I didn't have to tell them. They didn't want to get out of the car. I went into the house and said, 'My parents aren't going to come out. We're going to have to leave.'"

Ellen Kameya wasn't going to let the Kasais go. They had come this far and now sat in her driveway. She went out of the house, and for fifteen minutes she spoke to them while they sat in the car. Ellen shared Valerie's coming out story and talked about how she and Harold were "surprised and disappointed" and how "she understood that it would be a difficult life for her as a lesbian." After much coaxing, Mr. and Mrs. Kasai accepted her invitation to come into the house. To refuse such generosity would be rude, and above all, the Kasais cared about appearances.

Keith recalled that it was a small group that gathered at the Kameyas', maybe ten in all. He said, "Other people talked first, and then it came around to us. I talked for a while, and then they asked my father how he felt about what was going on." His father said something, but nothing substantive that Keith recalled. ("He kind of talked.") His mother didn't say anything at all but cried the whole time.

Despite this, Keith thought, "It was good for her [Mrs. Kasai] because she was probably holding all of this in. It was actually good for them to see that I'm not the only one." And the gathering being all Asian Americans (and the hosts, specifically Japanese American, like the Kasais) "made it easier." He said, "If they were White, it probably wouldn't have gone over well."

On the way home, his parents made no attempt to hide their displeasure at Keith's subterfuge. Keith remembered them saying, "I wouldn't have gone if I knew." But they also added, "They were so nice."

Their reconciliation was not complete overnight, but through the meeting at the Kameyas', Keith was able to show his parents what he couldn't have told them, or what they couldn't have accepted from him even if he could.

Despite efforts to de-gay AIDS, homophobia remained imprinted in the DNA of the virus. In her counseling practice at APAIT, Margaret found herself processing with her clients the homophobia they encountered from their biological families, especially at the end stage of the disease when the window of reconciliation shrank by the minute. She recalled a client, Michael, who came from a "pretty prominent" family in the Japanese American community. Michael had disclosed neither his sexual orientation nor HIV status to his parents:

> Everyone was different in their process. With Michael, it was anger, it was guilt, it was fear because he was alone, he didn't have a partner. It was regrets, so much that he hadn't done. That's where we started. He was entering the end stage of AIDS. He couldn't even talk to his parents about being sick because that meant he would have to tell them he was gay. I said, "Michael, how do you want to handle it? What would be the ideal situation for you?" He said, "I don't really want them to know. But maybe if they knew, then they'd understand. But I don't want to be a burden."

This is another illustration of the layers of cultural barriers to coming out, not only in the Asian American community, but perhaps also in other immigrant communities. Underneath all the familiar layers of shame, guilt, fear of rejection or violence, and possible loss, there is that expectation that we should not add more burden to our families when they were already so burdened by racism in the US.

Once Michael could acknowledge what he really wanted, Margaret took him on this journey one secure step at a time. Through this visioning process, Michael narrowed down that his parents and his sister were the most important people he needed to reconcile with before he passed, not the rest of the extended family. He was already close to his sister. They decided to engineer a group conversation "where he could just talk to his dad and his mom, feeling that his sister would be a strong advocate for him." Margaret helped Michael anticipate their reactions. Like Keith's family, Michael's parents were from Hawai'i. She said, "The father was pretty conservative, strong-willed. He would have the harder time. The mother would be like, 'Oh, my God. I don't know what's going on.'"

They even worked out where the conversations should take place (at the parents' home) and the sitting arrangement (Michael's sister sitting next to him). She explained, "I went the structural family therapy route, given the family dynamics." Structural family therapy focuses on changing the family structure to disrupt negative communication or interaction patterns among family members. After the first conversation, and with Michael's permission, Margaret started talking to his parents separately. Margaret recalled, "The family was so private that they asked me to come at night, after dark, because they didn't want people to see someone coming to the house and think there was a problem. It's that whole stigma thing again. How do you, knowing you have a short amount of time, help navigate that relationship in a way that the client is comfortable with it enough that he can go peacefully?" In other words, she had months to erase a lifetime of homophobia. She went through a similar process with the parents, focusing on what they wanted for their son. "The sister was really supportive, and that helped. Michael was pretty far along in the disease, so it sped up the process a little bit, especially for the father. Ultimately, he told Michael, 'You're my son no matter what.'"

They took Michael in and took care of him in his last days. The turnaround touched Margaret. "The father just carried him to the bathroom, carrying him like a baby. In the end, it was his son. He couldn't run from that. Part of it was Michael wanting to please his father, but feeling like he didn't live up to his expectations. So he projected, saying that his father would never understand. That wasn't the case. That was his perception of his father, this typical conservative, Japanese from Hawai'i, macho American guy. But he loved his son. I don't know if he was ever able to say that to Michael, but he definitely showed it in the end." Margaret choked up a little bit before she continued:

> He died at the parents' home. The day before he died, he was still in and out of consciousness. The parents called me and said he was going to go. I asked, "Do you think I can come talk to Michael?" They had wanted me to come. I asked him, "Michael, I think the end is pretty close. What do you want to tell your parents?" I wrote everything down. Then I told his parents, "This is what Michael shared with me. This is what he wants you to know." It was a lasting gift for them to know that. . . . I think they really appreciated it.

Margaret stayed at APAIT for less than two years. By the time Michael passed away, Margaret had left the agency to work at the Little Tokyo Service Center (LTSC), where she was promoted to director of social services in 2016. She went to Michael's funeral, where she ran into a coworker from LTSC who happened to be Michael's cousin. The coworker came up to her and said, "I didn't know you knew Michael. How did you know him?" Margaret responded vaguely, "Oh, he and I worked together at one time." The coworker pressed, "You worked at the phone company?" Trying to keep Michael's confidentiality to the very end, Margaret lied and said yes. Later she found out that Michael's parents told this cousin afterward that Michael had come out to them and Margaret had helped them with the grieving process.

In the end, Michael's parents claimed him as he was.

In the interview, after Margaret told me this story, we both reached for a tissue. She said, "I still talk about Michael how many years later? Thirty something years later, I still grieve. I feel bad for the parents. I'm sure it's really tough for them, but I did the best I could." I reminded her that Michael got to die at home, with his family around him, and more importantly, their knowledge and understanding of who he really was. It was huge, especially for someone who was initially skeptical she would have any impact on a population that she hadn't known much about. "I did the best I could" seemed to be an understatement.

To this, Margaret, true to her humble self, responded, "Yeah, I learned a lot."

To casual observers, AIDS was a biomedical movement. It was about finding a cure, getting medications to be approved, and battling pharmaceutical companies and health-care bureaucracy for access. People also remember AIDS for changing how we do public health in this country. The creative and often shocking ways to convince people to use condoms or to get tested were unprecedented. On both counts, these casual observers are not wrong.

However, AIDS activism touched me most, as a gay man of color who was just coming of age during the AIDS crisis in LA, in how it disrupted previous notions of what it meant to be both Asian and gay and encouraged the building of a viable community that was for us, by us. The disease raised our visibility because it forced many of us to come out to our families, sometimes in the most public of ways, and transfer the burden of recognition from us to those who claimed they loved us. Although some parents failed that test when it was put to them, many rose to the occasion and became advocates and allies. We didn't win over everyone, but enough came to our side to challenge the prevailing heterosexist norms.

By helping people like Keith and Michael confront the homophobia that hit home the closest, the AIDS work that Margaret and others did lifted the veil of silence for the rest of us—LGBTQ people in the Asian American community, regardless of our HIV status. Struggling with the homophobia in our "home" community was an important hallmark that made Asian American AIDS activism distinct. Militant AIDS activists at the time liked to disrupt Catholic masses to highlight the church's obtuse prescription against homosexuality or condom use. But Joël Tan would tell these mostly White activists that they'd have to go through him if they wanted to get in his grandmother's face in her place of worship. Joël wasn't overlooking the ostracization he felt from his "home" community, but he wanted to struggle with it on his own terms. Not fighting every battle but insisting on our place by those who don't love us perfectly is one strategy of cultural change. This work, no less revolutionary, was definitely more strenuous, and often heartbreaking.

CHAPTER 13

What AIDS Animated

Y OU COULDN'T FIGHT AIDS IN THE ASIAN AMERICAN COMMUNITY
without defusing homophobia. The social marketing campaigns, like
"Facing HIV and AIDS," did this in the broader ethnic immigrant communities. And the direct client work that the Asian Pacific AIDS Intervention Team (APAIT) staff, like Margaret Endo, did in trying to help
people with AIDS reconcile with their birth families accomplished this
on a more interpersonal level. Helping straight people understand and be
more comfortable with queer sexualities was just one side of the equa-
tion. Another strategy was to support LGBTQ-specific spaces in the
Asian American community so those who were now ready to come out
had a safe space to find each other and build their own network.

The mid-1990s witnessed a flourishing of LGBTQ Asian American
organizations in Southern California. Asian/Pacific Lesbians and Gays
(A/PLG), from which APAIT sprang, was founded in 1980, sort of the
grandfather to these organizations. And like some grandfathers, it was
becoming a little distant and irrelevant to the upstarts. A/PLG replicated the problematic racial-sexual dynamics of the gay men's community from that time. By the 1990s, young people who had been critical of
racism in the gay community were not drawn to A/PLG.

In 1984, the Gay Asian Rap Group (GARP) emerged in Long Beach
among college students and other young gay Asian men, offering an
alternative not only in its Asian-only membership policy but also in its
progressive narrative that did not place Asian men in a subordinate

position to White men, sexually or otherwise. A few years later, GARP formalized and became the Gay Asian Pacific Support Network (GAPSN). The women in A/PLG—very few to begin with, especially in its leadership—began to organize separately as well, first as Asian Pacific Lesbians and Friends (A/PLF), and later, in 1993, as Los Angeles Asian Pacific Islander Sisters (LAAPIS).

In the 1990s, LGBTQ Asian American organizing was becoming more ethnic specific. These immigrant organizations were outgrowing pan-ethnic organizations like LAAPIS and GAPSN that couldn't adequately address their needs. There were organizations for Chinese (Chinese Rainbow Association), Filipino (Barangay), Japanese (JUST), Korean (Chingusai), South Asian (first Trikone, then Satrang), and Vietnamese (Gay Vietnamese Alliance). Vietnamese queer women also formed Ô-Môi with a membership that, like the Gay Vietnamese Alliance, crossed both Los Angeles and Orange counties, but also included some trans men (a policy that was meant to accommodate early members who used to identify as lesbians). In 1994, the Japanese American Citizens' League (JACL), after some internal strife, became the first non-LGBTQ national civil rights groups after the American Civil Liberties Union to endorse marriage equality. Out of the organizing that made that victory possible, queer JACL members in Southern California convened an LGBTQ chapter. Continuing the activism that the Kameyas started when their daughter came out to them in 1988, they and other Asian American parents of LGBTQ children continued to organize, paving the way for the formation of the API Parents and Friends of Lesbians and Gays chapter in the San Gabriel Valley in early 2000s. In addition, a loose network of young queer Asian American college students emerged in the early 1990s that sometimes converged in these community spaces.

Some community leaders bemoaned what they saw as the fragmentation of the LGBTQ Asian American community and the possible diffusion of its influence, but many others understood this evolution as a signal of the emerging diversities—along ethnic, gender, and sexual lines—that the early pan-ethnic organizations could not readily absorb. Many of these ethnic-specific organizations were better at accommodating limited English proficient immigrants by offering programming and informal spaces in their respective native tongue. English was not presumed to be the dominant language, and assimilation was neither a starting point nor a desired destination. Though separately organized, these community groups convened under the aegis of the Asian Pacific Islander Pride Council to raise their visibility in both broader Asian American and LGBTQ communities. At the annual Pride parade in West Hollywood, Pride Council members marched as one contingent but each behind its distinct banner, showcasing both diversity and unity of the community.

APAIT leaders saw in this decentralization of community organizations an asset in outreach and education. These organizations provided their members a safe space to not only destigmatize their desire, but also to lift it up as the basis for a collective identity, often with a distinct sensibility that set it apart from the gay and lesbian mainstream. (Notice, for instance, that with the exception of GVA, these ethnic-specific groups eschewed the word "gay" or "lesbian" in their names.) The more vibrant the ethnic-specific organizations were, the more they would be able to bring together those immigrants who did not easily identify with the LGBTQ label, including that hardest-to-reach population, the holy grail of outreach: men who have sex with men (MSM). APAIT didn't just work with these organizations; it also built them up. As early as 1995, APAIT applied for funding to provide technical assistance and fiscal sponsorship to several of these networks in Korean, Filipino, Vietnamese, and South Asian communities. At the 1995 APAIT board retreat, Dredge Kang espoused a broader framework for HIV prevention that was consistent with the agency's approach to community building: "I envision that many of our programs will shift to modalities in which HIV prevention is an outcome rather than an activity." In other words, HIV prevention was not just condoms and testing anymore. He saw these community groups where LGBTQ immigrants could find each other and come out safely as part of this broader HIV prevention framework. Looking back, Dredge also recognized how AIDS partly fueled the explosion of queer Asian American organizations in the 1990s: "AIDS gave gay men, in particular, a platform that they had never had before. It was an issue that brought sympathy to the community. It was also an issue that the community organized against, and therefore, developed institutions around. We had new forms of credibility that didn't exist before."

APAIT cosponsored community events, like dances and film screenings, with these groups. Its staff conducted safer-sex education in their spaces and drew volunteers from them. The members from these ethnic-specific organization might even become HIV workers, and not just at APAIT. In the mid-1990s, Stephano Park found a job doing HIV outreach at Kheir, which was part of the Asian Pacific AIDS Education Project. Stephano had met Dredge at Chingusai, the Korean LGBTQ support group. Stephano said, "We were busy organizing Chingusai. [Dredge] and I became close very quickly. He became almost like my brother in a way." Stephano credited Dredge and others at APAIT as important resources at his new job.

According to Stephano, Dredge presented HIV education workshops to Chingusai members at "a social gathering or a slumber party at some-body's house." He said, "Dredge made it fun. He gave us some incentive items, and he asked questions." He thought Dredge was excellent in drawing interactions, but jokingly, like needling a brother, Stephano "gave him a hard time" when the presentation went a little long into the night. APAIT also provided some seed funding for Chingusai to install a "warm line" and a PO box for community members who wanted more anonymous communication. (As opposed to a hotline, a warm line does not have a person to pick up a call at any given moment, so the caller would have to leave a message and wait to be called back.) Stephano was typically the "responder" for the warm line, because of his leadership at Chingusai, his bilingual ability, and also his work at Kheir, where his manager allowed him to "conduct that duty while at work." According to him, the calls were mostly from closeted Korean lesbians and gay men who wanted to come out and find community. In this case, the resources from APAIT and Kheir allowed people living in the closet in the Korean community, men or women, immigrant or US-born, HIV positive or neg-ative, to find Chingusai more easily.

The explosion of the LGBTQ social groups powered ethnic-specific out-reach, especially in communities that had been marginalized by the pan-ethnic Asian umbrella. For instance, APAIT started a South Asian Outreach Task Force. Ghalib Shiraz Dhalla, one of the first South Asian staff members at the agency, found out about the job as he became involved in Satrang, the local LGBTQ South Asian social group.

Ghalib, an Indian gay man, immigrated from his birthplace of Kenya to the US in 1989, where he was "twice removed from the motherland." He enrolled in a program in graphic arts and marketing at Woodbury College in Burbank. Ghalib, who had been certain about his attraction to men since his teenage years, had come to the US by himself, untethered from his family. "I've always identified in my soul as a gay man," he said. "I felt like in order to grow, I had to cut the umbilical cord from my family. In LA, I would have the space to, as clichéd as it sounds, spread my wings. I was seduced by the image of LA or Hollywood, like so many who grew up in another part of the world. We grew up with these fantasies of America. I just felt like, 'That's where I can truly be myself.' That sounds kind of brave right now, but it was tough."

Not yet twenty-one, Ghalib had a hard time gaining entry into bars and clubs. And if one couldn't do that, one might as well be invisible in the gay community. At college, he met some gay men, but they were all in the closet. "I was grappling with so many other issues," he said. "Cultural shock, the fact that I sounded different because I had an accent." All of this made it hard for him to make friends. Ghalib's origin story was a reminder that West Hollywood was not for all gay men, and if HIV outreach and education were limited to these obvious gay enclaves, a lot of people who needed information and services would be missed.

Finally, in the mid-1990s, Ghalib "met one [gay] Indian person, and then another, and then it just evolved from there." One of these men was the late Mushtaque Jivani, who in 1997 was putting together Satrang with his network of friends. Ghalib went to a potluck at Mushtaque's home, apparently one of forty people at what would turn out to be the first Satrang meeting. From the beginning, Ghalib said Satrang leaders discussed the AIDS crisis with the membership because the silence around the epidemic in the South Asian community paralleled the denial of LGBTQ people. Ghalib said, "The tragic irony of the Indian community is that, like the Greeks, Indians actually make sex sacred. It's apparent in their temples, in their literature. So for the community not to talk openly about sex is a real tragedy. It goes back to the influence of the British. That's when all the laws [against homosexuality] were introduced. That's truly sad because they relegated that part of their culture to oblivion."

As an immigrant, Ghalib also discovered that the West's promise of sexual freedom was disappointingly empty. "I don't think we're a very sexually liberal country," he said. "We are a window-dressing sexuality. Maybe there was this era of debauchery and hedonism in the seventies and early eighties before AIDS took over. With AIDS, there is this ghostly sound in your subconscious that is always saying that you're gonna get punished for it, because that's what religion or society tells you. Every pleasure is inevitably spliced with guilt and the fear of retribution." Drawing a contrast with his home culture, Ghalib said that gay people in India "didn't have marches, and we didn't brandish rainbow flags, but the sex was everywhere. Maybe it was a dysfunctional type of sex because there was no acknowledgment of what was going on. Maybe decadence requires crimes of repression because people steal their pleasures with a little more desperation and hunger." Same-sex behavior, Ghalib insisted, was indigenous to Indian culture.

Through Satrang, Ghalib met Zul Surani, another Kenyan-born South Asian gay man who was also an Ismaili, a very progressive and esoteric Islamic sect Ghalib belongs to. Zul had just started the South Asian Outreach Task Force at APAIT. Probably because Ghalib was an immigrant who knew multiple Indian languages, Zul recruited him to work with him. Ghalib accepted the part-time job. "Honestly," he said, "I just wanted to stay involved with people that I could relate to. I don't know if it was as much activism as it was my way of being part of my community. AIDS was something we could do as a family."

Based on their personal experiences, Zul and Ghalib knew that the South Asian MSM that they needed most to reach would not be found in the streets of West Hollywood. "A lot of immigrants remain very secluded," Ghalib said. "They create a sort of nucleus almost and they don't go outside of it. Information is harder to penetrate that wall." Instead of the same venues that other AIDS organizations covered, they scoured LA County for its many gas stations and convenient stores, where many immigrant South Asian men toiled behind the counters. Stereotypical as it might sound, they felt that it was "an obvious choice" to find "people that came from certain social and economic strata that actually needed that type of education." "If you found an Indian person in a gay bar or a club," Ghalib continued, "certainly, that's an opportunity. Chances are, they're probably a little more educated about that stuff." Besides, gay bars and clubs were not where you would find a lot of queer South Asian men in the 1990s. He added, "If you saw one Indian out there in West Hollywood, you'd think you had witnessed a rebirth. It was astonishing. 'Oh my God, there's an Indian across the street. Let's run to him before he gets away!' I certainly recruited quite a few people and brought them into Satrang. I remember calling Rashmi [Choksey, a Satrang leader], saying, 'Give this guy a call. There's new meat in town.'"

Ghalib emphasized that the challenge was not limited to picking the right outreach venues:

> India has over twenty languages. Written, I would say more than a dozen scripts. That posed an enormous challenge. Just because you see somebody who looks Indian to you, doesn't mean they speak the same language. If somebody wanted to avoid having a conversation, it would be very easy for them to feign ignorance. Not to mention the fact that approaching them itself implied in the minds of the person we were talking to that we thought they were gay. There were times when they would just giggle and look at us like, "Oh, here come the gays." But more often they would think, "Why is he talking to me about all this? I'm not gay. I'm not bisexual. Yeah, I may have done something with another man, but what does that have to do with this [safer-sex] package he's giving me?" Remember in immigrant communities like ours, you can have an encounter with another man, it doesn't define you as gay or bisexual.

The distinction between the sexual acts and the sexual identity made these immigrant men think that AIDS would not affect them. It was why Ghalib thought the term *men who have sex with men*, while "just a ridiculous euphemism, frankly," was also "very academically necessary." It shifted the frame of who you would outreach to and how.

In a pair (never alone and three is a crowd), Ghalib and Zul (or sometimes volunteers they recruited from Satrang) would go into a store and wait until the staff was available. When they were not serving any customer, the pair would go up and introduce themselves. "It's like a sales job," said Ghalib:

> You ask them where they're from. You try and build a bridge, create a sense of affinity, and then you tell them what you're there to do. The fact that we look Indian would either make them suspicious or comfortable. It could go either way. I never used the word *gay* or *bisexual*, but just made it about the fact that there was a plague out

there and how they could avoid it. "You don't have to come clean to us about what you've been up to. If there is a chance that you're out there, here's something [a condom] you could use." Sometimes the answer was, "I'm married. I don't need this." In that case, I'd say, "Hold onto it and read it." Even if they were completely straight, they might know a brother or a cousin. The point is to make sure that the Indian community was protected from contracting HIV. You could have a really good encounter, or you could have one that was a complete disaster, and the guy screamed at you to get out. "What the hell are you doing giving me condoms?"

Ghalib actually found this uncertainty electrifying. "We were nervous," he continued. "We were brave. It was thrilling. It felt like we were making a difference and I think we really did."

On a good night, a few hours of outreach might yield five or six good conversations. But it wasn't just about AIDS. Ghalib and his crew "put themselves out there in a very vulnerable position" and laid bare the misperception that there were no LGBTQ people in their community. "We were taking a stand for our sexuality," he said. "Certainly, they couldn't say it's a White man's or American thing when you've got two Indians standing in front of you. I think that did shift their perception somewhat." Ghalib acknowledged that on its own, each encounter might not have a "dramatic" impact. But accumulated, this outreach project increased the visibility of LGBTQ people in the South Asian community. AIDS, Ghalib felt, "became the fertile ground on which we built not only the South Asian part of the APAIT organization, but also what is today Satrang."

The women at APAIT were also extremely active in the growing local queer Asian American women's community in the 1990s. When LAAPIS was founded in 1993, many of its leaders were already connected with APAIT in different ways. Unhei Kang was a LAAPIS cochair early on. So were Connie Wong, who served on the community advisory board at APAIT, and Shella Aguilar, who worked at PALS for Health. Connie said that "half the people who were on LAAPIS's board were also involved in APAIT. It's blurring now, whether something was through APAIT or LAAPIS." In our interview, Connie couldn't recall which involvement came first, though her partner, Heng Foong, reminded her that she was on both boards when they first met. The overlap in Connie's activist work was indicative of the flurry of community building activities that were taking place. Things were moving quickly, and they were still amassing warm bodies to push the work forward.

As part of her outreach to Asian American women, Unhei leveraged her leadership role at LAAPIS and conducted workshops at LAAPIS meetings, showing members how to have safer sex with Saran wrap and dental dams. "We also discussed the importance of cleaning sex toys, putting a condom on it, and essentially how to protect oneself and not transmit STD," she added. Unhei thought safer-sex skills were as relevant and practical to queer Asian American women as other workshops that LAAPIS offered, like "how to change your own tire." "Unhei made it fun," Connie recalled. "She made it like a dating game. It was education, but also socializing and networking. Even though Asian women, Asian lesbians, probably were the lowest of the lowest risk, there was this feeling that we needed to educate our sisters." Heng joined LAAPIS later than Connie—it was where they had first met and started dating. Heng remembered a safer sex workshop that took place at a different member's house, which meant that this workshop was offered more than once in this community space.

Both Unhei and Connie also remembered that APAIT, LAAPIS, and GAPSN would often cosponsor social events like dances and screenings of films with LGBTQ and Asian contents for the Los Angeles Asian Pacific Film Festival (organized by Visual Communications around late April and early May) or the Los Angeles LGBTQ Film Festival (organized by OutFest in July). More than creating a space where their members could enact a public racial and sexual identity, these community events also raised LGBTQ Asian American visibility in broader communities. In a city where LGBTQ Asian American community building was historically marked by gender segregation more often than not, the community response to AIDS provided an unprecedented opportunity for co-gender organizing. Beyond joint events, sometimes APAIT even dedicated their staff time to actually working on building these smaller and newer organizations.

Like many young queer activists who came into AIDS work in the 1990s, Diep Tran was politicized in college. She came out during her undergraduate years at the University of California, Riverside. "You took a class on postcolonialism, and it just fucked everything up," Diep said. "Then I had a class on sexuality. That was it. There was no way I wasn't going to come out at that point. I came out with a bunch of Asian American queers, too. It was intersectional before we learned that was a word." After college, she sought out APAIT. She explained, "I didn't want to work on AIDS per se. This was the time after Rodney King and the Thai garment workers in El Monte." The rescue of these workers held captive in an apartment complex exposed the slave-labor conditions and human trafficking that activists said had always marked the garment industry. It had radicalized many young Asian Americans. "I wanted to work on justice, through whatever door," Diep continued. "I wanted to work with an API organization for sure, and I wanted to work with potentially a queer organization. They [APAIT] were the only game in town. If you were an API queer, you'd already been to a club where they were passing out the safer-sex kits, and you'd seen the ads that were out. APAIT loomed large. It felt radical."

For a chance to be in that intersectional space and work with other Asian American queers, Diep took a part-time job at APAIT in late 1994, but doing something that was anything but radical. Because of its cultural competence with the Asian immigrant communities, APAIT received a subcontract to conduct sensitivity training to providers. Diep was their "cross-cultural trainer." "I hated the position," she said unequivocally. "The only people that were getting really great treatment were cisgender White gay men. Those were the people who had the best treatment, the best outpatient care, just a more complex and rich support network. Other people seeking services had to deal with homophobic providers or providers who had racist stereotypes. They would show up once [to an appointment], never showed up again or were just forgotten." The training supposedly taught providers to put aside their biases in working with people from different backgrounds. Developed by the agency that subcontracted APAIT, the curriculum tried to explain cultural differences, but Diep felt like they were "reiterating some stereotypes, like Asian Americans don't like to look you in the eye. . . . I was teaching people not to bow to an Asian American. After this eight-hour training, they'd think, 'We're good.' It's like, what the fuck? All I felt I was doing was coming in and making people feel better about themselves and then leaving and not having changed anything. It just didn't work for me."

When the subcontract was renewed, Diep asked Dean Goishi, her boss, if she could switch to another position. Dean assigned her to be the volunteer coordinator. Eventually, she also added women's programming to her job description. As part of her work, Diep worked on Ô-Môi—not *with,* but *on.* Already a leader in Ô-Môi, she was using APAIT time to plan events and produce newsletters for the support group:

> We just worked overtime all the time, so I never felt like I was short-shrifting [APAIT]. This organization was meant to serve the API community, and Ô-Môi was founded by Vietnamese dykes. If I did stuff that benefited Vietnamese dykes, bisexuals, lesbians and transgenders, I felt like that's fine. There were a bunch of organizations that say they served people with HIV, but they only served White men and they were fine with that. [APAIT] had such a small fraction of what APLA [AIDS Project Los Angeles] or the Gay and Lesbian Center had, I felt like my work was reparative justice.

To Diep, the AIDS movement was more than sickness and death:

> It wasn't just that people were dying, but it was also, people were dying and no one gave a shit because in the end the lives of gay men didn't matter. You can extrapolate that to the lives of any queer didn't matter. Compound that with the invisibility of Asian Americans, that just created such a lonely place for Asian American queers. Ô-Môi tackled that. I felt like we definitely created community and a culture that meant something. [Ô-Môi members] didn't have to go to a White gay club. They didn't have to go to a Vietnamese dancehall. It was substantial work. I felt like that was my true work, versus telling people about lube or standing outside of a club passing out safer sex kits. It's not that I didn't care about people with HIV, but [working on Ô-Môi] was what animated me.

According to Diep, Dean understood the significance of culture change and never pushed back. If nothing else, the work raised the

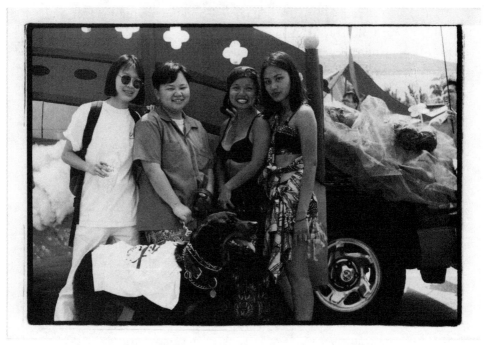

FIGURE 13.1. Gina Masequesmay (Ô-Môi member), Diep Tran (Ô-Môi member and APAIT staff member), Irene Suico Soriano (APAIT staff member), and Irene's cousin May, at the annual Pride Parade in the mid-nineties. Courtesy of Robert Berger.

agency's community profile. As she explained, "When we did interviews with *OC Register* about Ô-Môi, that linked directly to APAIT.

As Diep explained, APAIT "had a strong sense that if you build a strong [queer API] community, then that becomes a natural network for queer APIs with HIV." At a time when there was very little public or private funding for LGBTQ Asian American community building, AIDS money, which proliferated with the passage of the Ryan White CARE Act in 1990, became, in this vacuum, an engine for the growth of LGBTQ Asian American organizations in Southern California—yet another example of how taking on the toughest fights can lift up the broader community.

CHAPTER 14

The Dating Pool

ASIAN AMERICAN AIDS ACTIVISTS HAD A PERSONAL STAKE IN THE community that they were building; it wasn't just an abstract political project. The community relationships, while an asset for their work, were also personal ones. AIDS activism, Noel Alumit said, "gave us a sense of camaraderie. It really allowed us to come together and build those important relationships that help people develop. We had really important discussions about identity, who we were as gay Asian men. It helped us feel less alone, less angry."

"We were a very close agency," Tracy Nako added. "Even though I might be working Monday through Friday, on the weekends I would be at a bar or a bathhouse with the health educators, doing outreach and passing out condoms. It was never a nine-to-five job." Like Noel, Tracy was also looking for "camaraderie" as they quickly became immersed into this hard fight against the epidemic. He recalled that "many times after work, we would all go out, go to dinner, or hang out at each other's house." Some staff became roommates. They hung out so often that during the interview, Tracy thought he was once roommates with Dredge Kang (he wasn't; Dredge was a roommate with another APAIT staff member). The political/professional commingled with the personal/ social; or as Tracy described, "It was fluid. Your social life was all through your work life, and your work life was also your social life. It was an all-consuming type of job. You just couldn't shut it off."

Not to mention that all of these activists were in the prime of their sexual and dating life. These activists believed they were entitled to the inheritance of a transformative sexual revolution from the previous generation. As the US moved to the right politically with the ascent of the neoconservative Reagan/Bush regime, they fought even harder for it. There was no time to separate the fucking from the activism. The personal had never been this political. They had been telling others that they could have love (and just as importantly, good sex) even in the time of AIDS. They sang the gospel of "loving your Asian body" and pushed the "sticky rice" possibility as an alternative to the prevailing dominant racist hierarchy in the gay community. The dating pool for queer Asian men and women was getting bigger, thanks in part to all that community work through AIDS activism. Even the most restrained among these activists couldn't help but at least dip their toes in it.

Noel, who was in a relationship with a leader at the Gay Asian Pacific Support Network (GAPSN), remembered that APAIT staff had discussions about "professional standards" in fraternizing with the target population, guidelines that were more relaxed than those in most nonprofit organizations, including their parent agency, Special Service for Groups (SSG). "Back then," he said, "it was completely acceptable [for staff] to date a volunteer. That's why we were coming together. Even outreach. Theoretically we could sleep with somebody if we outreached to them. It was that loose. We'd have these really important discussions."

Noel wasn't being caustic at all when he said that these discussions were "important." Sexual and romantic relationships were not frivolous in the time of AIDS. Being able to love (and fuck) whomever you wanted was the fuel for AIDS activism, and the policing of desire was exactly what the more radical AIDS activists were fighting against.

Noel continued:

Hello, I'm a gay guy. I like other Asian guys. I'm outreaching to them, so I can't date these people? I was a member of Gay Asian Pacific Support Network. I was there as their friends. Or I could also be a professional doing a workshop for GAPSN. So where was that line drawn when I could and couldn't date them? That was a very blurry line. And then there were some situations where it did get really dicey. Like we were at an outreach, someone would say, "See that guy over there? Do not outreach to him. I really like that guy. I think he's really cute."

In that example, the staff ended up not reaching out to this person, so that they could approach him when the official outreach was over to ask him out. To guard against these "dicey" situations, the agency reached a compromise. According to Noel, staff had to wait two weeks before they could date or have sex with a community member they had outreached to. The staff did draw a very strict line when it came to clients. There was no two-week rule; staff-client romantic relationships were prohibited.

In a predominantly gay male space, the gay Asian men at APAIT definitely had their share of action. There were at least two instances where two gay male staff began a relationship. APAIT provided equal opportunities for some queer Asian women, too. Connie Wong and Heng Foong, for instance, might not have met directly at APAIT, but AIDS remained a constant background in their early courtship. Connie served on APAIT's advisory board, and Heng managed the PALS for Health program that collaborated often with APAIT staff. From their distinct vantage points, they saw Dean Goishi very differently. Connie thought he was a "warm teddy bear," whereas to Heng, Dean for many years felt like an "enigma." It wasn't until she went on an out-of-town work trip with Dean, when he revealed a lot more about his personal life, that Heng saw him beyond his role as "the director of APAIT, this really important fella." Still, he was never a "warm teddy bear" to Heng. No matter how differently they saw him, Dean and APAIT remained an integral part of their relationship, both professionally and personally.

Yet the coupling that challenged SSG's fraternization policy didn't come from APAIT's queer staff. That relationship had a rom-com beginning; that is, it did not begin well. Karen Kimura remembered her first encounter with JJ Joo this way: "One of my first tasks [at APAIT]—just because I was promoting HIV testing—was trying to find out who provided HIV testing in the community. I was just calling everybody, API, gay, whatever." Karen was used to getting cold shoulders on these cold calls. "Some people didn't want to talk to me at all." One day, she reached the Koryo Health Foundation, which housed a teen clinic in the Korean American community, and JJ took the call. "He was so rude to me," Karen recalled. "I thought, 'Who is this Korean guy? I'm just trying to get information.'"

JJ didn't remember the encounter at all. Prior to that call, he had been incorporating AIDS in his work, even when his job had not called for it. As the artistic director of the Asian American Community Teen Theater, he was "directing and writing pieces about substance use, tobacco use, gang intervention, HIV and AIDS, and STD." Later, at the Korean Youth Center (before they became the Koreatown Youth and Community Center), JJ "invited Noel and Unhei to present to our high school peer educators on specific issues impacting gay/bi issues in the Asian community. There weren't a lot of HIV/AIDS cases that we knew of in the Korean American community. We needed to educate the community."

By the mid-1990s, JJ's more progressive view on the epidemic, especially in a more mainstream Asian American community-based organization, caught the attention of the APAIT staff. JJ was invited to APAIT's open house. "That was the first time I actually saw the office," he said. "I knew Tracy and Dredge because I would see them at community events. And they said, 'JJ, we're hiring.' We chatted a bit about the position at the open house. It was a brand-new pilot project targeting API community called 'prevention case management.' I had heard about case management intervention for treatment programs [for people who already had AIDS, what Tracy had been doing at APAIT], but this was targeting HIV-negative or seropositive community." Prevention case management was an innovation in the mid-1990s in the HIV/AIDS field; more intense than prevention efforts, it was an early intervention for high-risk individuals and for people who were newly diagnosed to keep them from getting sick. JJ was intrigued. He went to a more formal second interview.

When Tracy and Dredge told Karen that they were about to hire JJ, she thought, "JJ Joo. Hmm. That sounds familiar." And when they told her his work experience in the Korean community, instead of being impressed, Karen realized, "Oh, yeah. That was the guy who was rude to me." That didn't keep him from getting the job. At APAIT, JJ managed a team, including future APAIT division director, Jury Candelario.

It didn't take long for JJ to correct Karen's misgivings about him, and they started dating. "At the time, we did have one rule," Karen said. "There was to be no dating on all levels. I'm sure it was broken. I knew I wasn't the first one. But I did have this tremendous guilt because I was part of management at APAIT." "But we weren't reporting to each other," JJ carefully pointed out.

"I just felt horrible because I was breaking our policy," Karen continued. "We're trying to keep it on the down low. I was just so worried and stressed out about this." Since a few close friends at APAIT already knew about their relationship, Karen felt "compelled" to "come clean" to Dean. When she finally revealed her transgression, she was surprised and thoroughly touched by Dean's response. "He was so overjoyed. He was so sweet." Karen still remembered to this day what he said: "If something so positive can happen out of this epidemic, if you can find love from this agency, I'm so happy for you."

Dean being Dean, he quickly remembered his role as the agency's director. Karen could tell he was back to his "practical" mode, ruminating on the dating policy that had stressed Karen out in the first place. He told Karen he would talk to the SSG board about the policy. Karen said that "they actually ended up going into this whole discussion, reviewed the policies, realizing that it was not a legal policy that they could enforce. They ended up changing it." AIDS work blurred the boundaries of personal and political, in perhaps more intimate ways than other movements, but it wasn't without a touch of irony that a heterosexual couple were the ones who opened up the space for all.

Though rightfully convinced that they weren't doing anything unethical, JJ thought a couple working in the same place couldn't be good for the relationship. He explained, "It's just awkward. You don't want to bring that home." He left the agency after two years and went to the county office that provided much funding for APAIT, becoming a contract monitor. Though he didn't leave the agency explicitly because of the relationship, he wondered if "maybe subconsciously that was on my mind."

His job at APAIT didn't last, but the relationship did. It still thrives. JJ and Karen have been married for years and live in the South Bay of LA County with their two children (figure 14.1).

Even as AIDS activism widened the intimacy possibilities for many, the epidemic continued to make dating harder for some who were living with HIV. Gay men were not immune to AIDS prejudice. Ric Parish instituted his own protocol to shield himself from disappointment. The

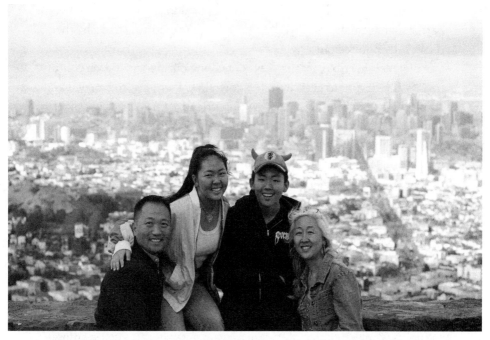

FIGURE 14.1. Karen Kimura Joo and JJ Joo, with their children, Kennedy and Nicholas, in San Francisco, 2019. Courtesy of JJ Joo.

first date was to check out the other person; there was no need to reveal his status. "If I made it to the second date, I would make it a point to always disclose because it's so much easier" than having be an issue when he went too deep into the relationship. Sooner or later, he just found it the easiest "to find other HIV-positive guys and get that out of the way, and not have it as an issue."

Many HIV-negative activists learned to get over their blinders. Tracy Nako remembered that the HIV-positive people he had dated were "shocked" that he was open to sero-different relationships. He said, "It was because of all my experience being in Los Angeles back in '93 or so, dating mostly men of color at the time and just assuming that the other person I met was positive because of the high incidence [rate]. If I had discriminated, I would not have a lot of people to date. I just assumed everybody was, and we'd just have to practice safe sex, anyway."

While at Kheir, Stephano Park also began dating someone who was HIV positive. He said, "I wasn't really afraid of the disease by then.

All the myths regarding the disease had been dispelled already. I was teaching people about it. . . . I knew I shouldn't hold that against him because it was really nobody's fault. I tried to be as normal as possible about it, too."

But the burden of normalcy fell harder on his HIV-positive partner:

> He was trying really hard to hide any type of symptoms or physical manifestation caused by HIV, so that I didn't have to think about it, so that it wasn't in my face. He was very careful whenever we had sex. He was taking the medication, but never in front of me. I had to ask him about his viral load every time he got the blood test. Even when he was feeling [sick], he wouldn't tell me. I think at some point he was throwing up and having adverse reactions [to the medication]. He tried to normalize everything, so that I wouldn't be reminded that there was this in the room.

Stephano understood that his partner's "insecurity" was "what he thought he had to do to keep the relationship going," despite Stephano's assurances that he could handle it. If the partner had a cold, he would be paranoid that Stephano would catch it from him., "He was more vulnerable to catch something from me," Stephano said. "But he'd say, 'I don't mind. I'll just suffer through.' It was kind of sweet." But also "bitter," he added. AIDS was such a big part of their lives that hiding it unwittingly prevented them from getting closer to each other. After about a year, they parted ways.

Dean was right. Even in those times when a community was most distressed, when grief was always a shadow, love and joy were not luxuries, but necessities. But make no mistake, it was a plague war. There were plenty of casualties—among clients, and even staff. The narrators did not always invoke their names in the interviews. After all, while the dead had never left them, many had put away this grief for years. But these spirits, once manifested in their words, were palpable.

CHAPTER 15

Good Grief

DEAN GOISHI COULDN'T CONFINE THE EPIDEMIC TO JUST HIS professional life. The virus had so ambushed his generation of gay Asian men that the healthy ones, like Dean, often took on the caregiving responsibilities when they had any time away from their activism. While a director at the Asian Pacific AIDS Intervention Team (APAIT), he and his partner Tom Callahan took care of their friend Sidney, who had played an instrumental role in Dean and Tom getting together in 1991.

"[Tom and I] met at Cuffs," Dean said. He stopped to check if I knew that bar. Oh, yes, a small leather bar in pre-gentrified Silverlake, where I had lived as a young man in the 1990s. I recalled entering the bar through a gauntlet of men mostly older than me. Men were packed in so tight that it blurred the distinction between brushing against and groping. Before you could even see the bar in the middle of the establishment, you were greeted by The Principal, a pudgy regular in a leather vest prone to giving the patrons a jolly spanking. Even as the bar got darker the further you went in, you could still hear people making out or even more. Dean summed it up: "It's a raunchy bar!"

Knowing that I understood the setting, Dean continued. "They got closed many times by the health department. The neighbors complained because people would have sex outside. Tom and I met there. We ran into each other and I saw all the red flags: don't get involved with him; he's bad news."

"Because you met him at Cuffs?" I asked.

He nodded.

I couldn't tell if he was being sardonic. Even now, in their retirement—Dean was in his mid-seventies when I interviewed him, and Tom was almost ten years younger—the couple had an easy banter between them, even when it was mostly Dean needling Tom about something and Tom deflecting it with a self-deprecating joke. I pushed a little and said, "But *you* were at Cuffs."

He smirked and said, "I was only there because it was my neighborhood bar. I was sitting there, minding my own business. He was the one who approached me, but we did not exchange phone numbers."

Dean returned to Cuffs, his neighborhood bar, the following week. Lo and behold, there was Tom again. They talked a little more, but once again, they "left separately and did not exchange phone numbers." But in their conversation, they had talked about Tom's friend, a Japanese American named Sidney—"not a common name for a Japanese American," Dean pointed out. When Dean mentioned that he might know the same person, Tom called Sidney afterward and got Dean's number from him. Knowing that Sidney and Tom had had a tryst didn't make Dean any more eager to accept Tom's advance. Dean being only the second Asian American he had ever dated, Tom balked at the "rice queen" label: "I had two grains of rice!" The first date took almost a month to plan (mostly because of Dean's work schedule), but learning more about Tom helped Dean get over his initial reservation.

In 1995, when Sidney, who was HIV positive, fell "so ill that he couldn't stay at home," Dean and Tom, already cohabitating, took him in. Since Tom was a nurse, he took over much of the medical aspects of the caregiving. "Sidney was afraid of what the care was costing," Tom explained. "He was on Ensure, but I was able to get that for free because I knew the vendors. I did his IVs at home. When Sidney fell ill, he started to put up walls. I think he was embarrassed and a little bit scared. He wanted to go home, too, but it was easier for me to take care of him if he lived with us. Otherwise, I would never be home."

Sidney's situation did not improve after a few months, prompting Dean to call Sidney's sister in Hawai'i to pay a visit. Sidney passed away in the hospital while she was there. "If he could just hang on for a few more months," Dean said, "we could've probably gotten him the cocktail."

Sidney was not the only one Tom had taken care of and lost. Right before Sidney, another ex, Bob, also got sick. Tom recalled that "when [Bob] was in the convalescent home, every day after work, I would stop by and pick up all his dirty clothes—because you'd have a lot of those, with accidents and stuff—and bring them home, wash them, then bring them to work with me so I could drop them off after work and pick up new dirty ones and do it all over again." A former corporate executive, Bob had amassed enough wealth to allow him to live his last days and die at home, as he wished. Tom was the one who made the arrangement for round-the-clock nurses. Unfortunately, Bob died the day Tom was ready to bring him home. After his death, Tom executed his will, and his family from Minnesota was so grateful that they compensated him for his role as the executor, even when Bob's will had stated that Tom would serve without a fee.

Just months apart, Tom lost two good friends whom he had taken care of until their death. Dean thought that was why Tom became reluctant to go to anyone's funeral. The way Tom took care of his friends, though, reassured Dean that he had made the right choice for his life partner. For someone who prided himself on his instincts, on being a good judge of character, Dean had been wrong about Tom's being the trouble he didn't need.

Tom also spoke of Dean's accomplishments with the same twinkle in his eye, gushingly to make up for Dean's humility. "I was always amazed and awed," Tom said:

> Whenever we met new people, even my family, they'd say, "What do you do?," and he would always say, "Oh, I work for an AIDS organization in the Asian Pacific community." You know, like no big deal. Then I'd go, "Wait, wait, wait. When I first met you, you were a volunteer working to establish what became APAIT. Then he started getting grants and funding, spent hours and hours working on it." I always told people, "He went from being a half-time person to having twenty-plus employees in a building downtown." I was very proud.
>
> He was on the president's council on AIDS or some boards or another. He would go to the CDC and NIH. He was involved in this seminar or that seminar, speaking on this and that. I'd tell people, "To really know what he did, Google his name." Back in the old house in

LA, the office had more wall space, and it was just covered with commendations, appreciation, all kinds from the city, from the county, the state, the federal government. He was a mover and shaker.

Tom took a small breath before saying it again. "I was very proud."

When it comes to the AIDS movement, one cannot divorce love from grief. So many gay male relationships like Dean and Tom's were fortified in the frontlines against AIDS. Their intimacy, in turn, fueled Dean's longevity in AIDS work. Dean said, "Tom's support kept my head above water. You cannot underestimate the value of knowing somebody would pop me up when I was down."

When Gil Mangaoang revealed his positive status to Juan Lombard, the news, which would've broken many heteronormative marriages, only steeled their resolve in not only their relationship, but also their AIDS work.

Juan's reconciliation had its roots in a long history dealing with AIDS all around him. His younger brother George had died of encephalitis, an AIDS-related complication, when George was only twenty-eight. George had visited Juan and Gil when they were still living in the Bay Area. Fresh out of high school, he wasn't out to either of them yet, but Gil "knew George was gay from the first time I went to visit his family. My gay-dar was working." While visiting them, George invited Gil to go out to talk, without his brother. "I already knew what that talk was going to be," Gil said. "He asked me, 'What do you think Juan is going to say?' I said, 'I think he's going to be so happy he's got a gay brother.'"

"I was, that's true," said Juan, who took over the story from there. Active as a volleyball player, George was competing in a Gay Olympic tournament the next time he was in San Francisco. Juan got to experience the opening ceremony, where the crowd was cheering the players as they marched in. George had looked up to Juan all his life, but at the moment, Juan the older brother felt a new sense of pride and admiration. "He was a handsome guy," Juan said. "When I went home to New Orleans, we would go to the gay bars. It was mostly White; that's just the way the city was organized. But everybody knew him. He would introduce me. 'This is my brother.' It felt like, wow. It was just so nice how he treated me." It made Juan feel like he was with royalty.

AIDS took George quickly. "By the time he told me he had HIV, his T-cells were down to ninety or something. It was really low. I figured he didn't have much time. I asked him if he wanted to come out to California. He said no. He wanted to stay in New Orleans." When George slipped into a coma, Juan made the tough decision not to go to New Orleans. There was nothing he could do, and as Gil said, "That's not the last memory you want to have of someone." Juan said, "You feel a certain loss when you have someone who was special that you couldn't replace. I miss him a lot. There were experiences we could've had that got lost."

His brother's death was partly why Juan, newly trained as a nurse by the time he moved to LA, went to work in the AIDS ward in the county. I don't want to romanticize the heroism here. The truth is, working with people with AIDS at the last stages of the disease could just as easily aggravate the grief as alleviate it. "I watched young, beautiful guys in their twenties"—like his brother—"who would be gone in two weeks," Juan said. "It was just awful." Juan did bedside care:

> People would have so much diarrhea. It was just cruel. Or they had lung problems and they couldn't breathe. I'll never forget this one guy. He was an immigrant from Mexico. His family didn't know and he was by himself. They were asking him if he wanted the ventilator. And he asked me because no one was there to help him. I said, "I don't think it's the best thing for you because it's not going to save you. And it's a horrible way to go." When you're on the ventilator, you can't breathe yourself and they give you so much drugs. It's cruel.

Even though he was HIV negative, Juan was intimate with the disease long before Gil became infected. Neither of them remembered the exact conversation when Gil revealed his status. Gil knew he was full of "remorse" for "bringing more grief into a relationship." Juan didn't know which emotion came first, but disappointment was one of earlier ones. Not so much disappointment at Gil, although I'm sure there was some of that, but disappointment that the plague had caught up with them when he thought they, then in their forties, were safe from it. "I thought we had escaped that," he said. "Haven't we paid enough? How much more do we have to give up for it? There is a certain part of me that understands this is part of what the community has to go through. It's something that happens all the time. We all have to be a part of it." This was why he didn't run away. In fact, he plunged toward it, head first, with his true love. Gil was told he had no more than seven years ahead of him. In spite of that, the couple put a down payment on a condo in the Silverlake neighborhood, where they held their marriage ceremony, and moved forward with their homemaking plans.

Sally Jue said that early in the epidemic, some gay men "referred to HIV as 'our disease.'" Why would anybody want to call this their disease? Why would anybody want ownership of that? "I think they were grieving a loss," she reasoned. "They were part of this community of grief, and they were able to build something different and special which united them in a more meaningful way that is more than just sex and bathhouses. Being gay wasn't just defined by having sex with other men." When Sally explained how that grief had become synonymous with gay men's identity, Juan's decision to stay with Gil made a lot of sense to me. AIDS would always be part of who that first afflicted generation was, even for those who were HIV negative.

Over the years, Gil and Juan's relationship went through multiple non-heteronormative phases—in what some might argue led to Gil's infection—but Juan was adamant that their relationship was just as solid, if not more so, than most heterosexual monogamy, precisely because of how the two survived the epidemic together. Years ago, Juan's father announced that he had made a planned financial gift to each of Juan's siblings' exes, but he had nothing for Gil. "I really got upset about it," Juan recounted. "I said, 'No, you're not going to do that unless you give something to Gil. How could you give something to my brother's ex that he doesn't like? My sister was left by this guy, and he's getting a gift? I'm staying with a guy who has HIV and we're going through all this stuff. And you're ignoring this?'"

While Juan toiled in the AIDS ward, Gil was working at APAIT. Because they had made a conscious decision to have the epidemic in their lives—at home and at work—they were very mindful about how not to let the virus invade and take over their lives. It didn't mean they grieved together. Gil said that "[Juan] would come home when he had one of those tragedies. Sometimes he wouldn't tell me, but I could tell that something happened at work."

"I saw so much of it," Juan added despondently.

Gil said, "I kept it separate mainly because a lot of the experiences you have to keep confidential. I loved my job because it was just part of who I am. It was a rewarding experience to know that I was helping someone, a privilege, but I couldn't divulge any details to Juan."

Juan said, "Well, I'd feel it."

"You have to survive," Gil continued. "You have to cut it off and say, 'It's behind that door. I'm leaving it there. I'm home now.' Otherwise, you go crazy."

The couple developed a wordless system of coping with grief. Their condo was on the top floor of a three-story building. At the end of a work-day, they would ascend to the rooftop deck. "We saw the entire city," said Gil, his hand moving expansively before him to indicate the panorama. "We had a 270-degree view. On a clear day, we could see Catalina [Island]." Juan added, "The sunset blew us away." "Oh my God," Gil followed, "it's sunset and the city is aflame."

Juan said, "Then I could at least go to sleep. I didn't have to take anything to fall asleep, because it was just so peaceful."

"It's like a different world," Gil interjected.

"You were away from the battlefield," Juan continued. "You could have some distance from it. You had to have some kind of tension releasing sources because you couldn't get through this stuff without it."

To manage their relationship while keeping their proximity to the AIDS crisis, Tom and Dean adopted different coping strategies with grief and stress, mostly based on their different upbringing. For Dean, it was his Japanese Buddhist heritage; for Tom, his Irish Catholicism. For Dean, the Japanese concept of *shikata ga nai*—"it can't be helped"—governed much of his reaction to the death and dying around him. The cultural concept reflects the Buddhist acceptance of suffering in this life. It wasn't resignation, though, as some people mistakenly think. If it was that, Dean wouldn't have ratcheted up his leadership responsibilities in the AIDS community over the years. This feeling was often counteracted by the notion of communal expectation, that they needed to do something for others who were not as fortunate. The more people became affected and the tougher the grief, the harder Dean worked. "It's just a fact of life for us," Dean said. "It was just the behavior that we thought was expected. I don't know if it is a coping mechanism."

Tom's coping strategies were full of ambivalence. On the one hand, there was tremendous survivor's guilt, perhaps traceable to his Catholic upbringing. "I was really upset when both [Sidney and Bob] died," he said. "To this day, I think, 'Why me? Why did I get off scot-free? Why didn't I have it?' They were nice people, they worked hard, they were smart. They were kind. Yet they're dead and I'm not." On the other hand, he said, "being Irish, there's no way you'll just say, 'It's just the way it is.' You want to punch somebody out." What placated his guilt and anger was his professional calling as a nurse. "Once you've been up on someone's bed and pounding their chest and they don't make it, there's a reality you become aware of." Although they tried to stay out of each other's grieving process, Tom did eventually absorbed, if only by osmosis, some of that *shikata ga nai* spirit. "There is a tranquility in just knowing it's nobody's fault," he said. "It just happened. I learned from that."

The detachment was not possible for many staff members who worked with clients directly. Pauline Kamiyama described taking a client home to Hawaiian Garden during the El Niño season of LA in the mid-1990s: "I drove a Toyota Tercel. No matter how fast the windshield wipers were going, I still couldn't see the road." Under the heavy rain and being unfamiliar with the directions (this was before GPS), Pauline was deathly afraid that she, not AIDS, was the one who would kill the client. All she could do was think about how to get him home. Staff members like Pauline felt personally responsible for the clients. "We did things that traditional mental health service providers wouldn't do," she said. "We crossed the line because we had to. We got rid of those boundaries in order to build trust. Every time we lost a client, it was just too much. You couldn't leave it at work. That was the down side of not having those clinical protocols and boundaries."

She organized a celebration of life for each client who passed as part of the dayroom activities and kept a scrapbook for each death. She acknowledged that it was good for the clients to have this grieving process with the staff. "It showed that we cared for them. They weren't just a number to us or a box to be checked off. It gave people comfort in knowing that they weren't just going to some random clinic." After one too many memorials, the accumulation of grief became overwhelming, and she had to leave APAIT. She explained, "We talked about self-care all the time. If you couldn't take care of yourself, you were no good to the clients. At a certain point, I needed to go."

It was even harder emotionally on staff when their HIV-positive coworkers fell ill. As a case manager, Tracy Nako felt it more than most. He said, "We had coworkers that ended up becoming my clients. They were my family in a way. There were no boundaries."

Yet the work that these sick staff members had been responsible for now—and which still had to be done—fell to the coworkers, who were burdened not only by grief for a friend dying, but also by the work stress of having to keep the programs going. Noel Alumit recalled:

> We would try to keep that job open as long as possible in case that person might come back, but we'd still have to do the work, while going through the psychological stress of knowing that this staff person was unavailable. It could be months. And sometimes, I'd be angry because we had to reach thousands of people, per our contract, and we were all struggling for numbers. Part of the frustration was that we worried that the quality of the outreach education wasn't as good, because we were talking to people really fast. We couldn't have deep and meaningful discussions with people.

Dean struggled a bit to understand how his staff was dealing with death and grief. *Shikata ga nai* didn't really work for the staff. Part of it was generational. The other part was that after a few years, the staff had grown to a point where the staffing structure had a layer of middle management. As a result, Dean had less face time with each person who worked at the agency. He relied on other staff to get an accurate read on staff morale. In the brief time that Margaret Endo Shimada was there as a counselor, Dean asked her to reach out to staff members who he thought weren't doing well. Margaret said that "Dean wasn't a warm and fuzzy person to everybody. Even though he might not have shown it, he always wanted to make sure the staff was okay."

"The regret I have is, I did not pay enough attention to the welfare and mental health of the employees, in making sure they did not burn out," Dean acknowledged. "I was probably naïve, idealistic, in thinking that if I could do it, my staff could do it, too." Noel said, "At first we had no bereavement process. There was no grief counseling. Someone would die, and we just ate it." It was clear that the staff needed an outlet.

Noel continued, "Dean could be pretty hard-nosed about it, about making sure that our contracts were doing well, that our numbers were met. The work could not stop was the problem. I was emotional, and one of the ways I acted out was I would question him a lot. 'Why are we doing these things? Why are we moving forward like this?'" Noel remembered "butting heads" with Dean to the point where Dean would pull him into his office.

Some staff members had a chance to see a softer side of Dean. Pauline remembered his going with her and other staff to a client's home to clean it before the client came back from a hospital. "It was overrun with cockroaches. Dean just quietly picked up a garbage bag and cleaned up the apartment with the rest of us. His compassion just stayed with me to this day," she said, amid sobs.

Over time, Noel said, "Dean got better about making sure that counselors would come in to talk to us." Sally Jue was one of them. Noel continued:

Dean used to get mad at us because we would spend lots of time putting together safer-sex kits. Thousands of safer-sex kits had to leave our office. Hours and hours and hours of opening a packet, putting a condom in there, and then the lube. Everyone would do that. It wasn't just the outreach team. Dean would get frustrated with us. "Can't you get volunteers to do this?" He thought that was a waste of our time, until a bereavement counselor came in and pointed out that that kind of repetition, and the camaraderie of coming together, talking about our day, bonding—but especially the repetition—was something that we could count on, we had control over. It was safe. It was routine. The ritual of putting these packets together was actually psychologically beneficial for us. After the bereavement counselor explained that, Dean never bothered us about that again.

Noel said that Dean understood this ritual was part of a "healing" process against the ongoing "uncertainty and impermanence."

And nowhere was this resolve for a healing culture tested more than the passing of one of their own, James Sakakura.

CHAPTER 16

This Darkness Is Not Your Life

JAMES SAKAKURA WAS BORN IN 1958; HE WAS THE THIRD OF PATRICIA Sakakura's four children. Mark, James's oldest brother (and at one time my dentist), arranged the interview I had with Patricia in 2018. She was almost eighty-eight then. Patricia met James's father when she attended the University of California, Berkeley, after World War II. The postwar boom fueled by the aerospace industry brought the Sakakuras to Southern California. The father found a job at Douglas Aircraft in 1956. Mark was born a year before they moved. "I was part of the luggage from San Francisco to LA," Mark quipped.

The Sakakuras settled in Gardena. Toyota Motors, where Patricia worked, was headquartered there. Both Mark and Patricia described a fairly typical suburban life, Japanese American style. They went to the Gardena Baptist Church, where the kids also attended Sunday school. Mark was very active in the Boy Scouts. "The infamous Troop 719," Mark said proudly of the Japanese American troop that was established in 1956, now one of the youth programs at the Gardena Valley Japanese Cultural Institute (formerly Moneta Gakuen, a Japanese language school founded in 1912). At his father's insistence, he also took judo classes at the local YMCA. Mark kept up the practice into his adult life. "I was a samurai," he said. "I was supposed to be tough." This revelation surprised me. Mark was my favorite dentist. His gentleness, a cool (young) uncle's vibe, was reassuring, a rare trait in his profession. It was hard for me to imagine him in a judo gi. "I was the kid that just liked to watch the clouds float by," he added. "I was easygoing, not much you'd like to see in a firstborn samurai." That made better sense.

With both parents working, Eileen, the second oldest, became, in Patricia's words, "the mommy" who looked after James and Cyrus, the youngest. Mark remembered James as "real curious, always asking questions," while his mother described him with adjectives like talkative, outgoing, and friendly. In high school, Mark said, "James had a super diverse group of friends. They included the kids that everybody looked down on. He had a circle of friends that were girls. The prettiest girls everybody's drooling over. 'Hey, that's the prettiest girl in school, and James just got a ride home from her.' He could maneuver in that environment, too."

If Mark was laid back, James could be a little intense.

Patricia recalled that "James and Cyrus were always at each other. One time, Cy went and wore one of Jamie's white jeans. When he found out, he was furious. When Cy came home, he punched him and told him, 'You're not supposed to be wearing my clothes.' He gave Cy a bloody nose, so Cy took off his jeans and wiped his nose with them. He threw them at Jamie and said, 'Okay, I won't wear your pants anymore.'"

Mark went to USC, and Eileen to Cal State Long Beach. James was accepted at UC Irvine, but the family couldn't afford to send a third child to college. Luckily, a relative helped James pay for his fees at UC Irvine. Even though Irvine wasn't that far from Gardena, they didn't see James for long stretches of time.

Out of the blue, Patricia and her husband received an invitation from James to meet in "J-Town" (Little Tokyo). At this meeting, James came out to his parents.

"My husband was furious," Patricia recalled. "He told James, 'I hate you, you no good son. You're not my son. I could kill you.' So Jamie took off. I had to listen to my husband rant and rave about that. It just made me so mad at him for not even worried about James. It [my resentment] kept growing and growing. I told him, 'I don't wanna even be married to you if that's the way you're gonna treat your child.'"

James was planning to tell his siblings next. Mark said, "After he talked to our parents, we knew something was going on. He came over to talk to us; Cy, Eileen, and I. My dad came into the room and just went berserk. He started physically abusing James. I had been in judo for fifteen years by then. I literally picked him up and threw him across the room. I told him, 'Don't you ever touch him again.' My dad had some unresolved issues about anger and authority. He's the oldest. He had to have everything his way, and everybody had to see things the way he did."

Mark knew his father expected him, the eldest, to aspire to this toxic form of "toughness." Patricia remembered that if Mark didn't do what her husband wanted him to do in judo class, he would throw Mark around until he was in tears. And he would say, "This is how you learn. This is how you gotta be." She said that "the younger kids would just watch in terror when [their father] threw [Mark] around." Mark attributed his father's toxic masculinity to "deep emotional scars" from a troubled childhood, where his father's mother "tortured him mentally with her words relentlessly." "He was trying to protect himself in his world," Mark reasoned. "Unfortunately, he couldn't bring himself to change. It was very sad." In Gardena, the siblings shared one room that was only big enough to hold a bunk bed, a crib, and one dresser. "We had a drawer a piece," Mark remembered. His youngest brother, Cy, would sleep in the crib until elementary school. "If his friends were gonna come over, he'd clean everything up and put a blanket over the crib, so nobody knew he slept in a crib still." In such overcrowded conditions, his siblings would pretend to be asleep in their room during one of their father's violent episodes with Mark, "but everybody would ask if I was okay when I came to bed," Mark said. This tension made him feel "much more alienated than [he] would like to have been to [his] siblings."

But when it mattered most, Mark became James's biggest advocate, turning the same toughness that was forced upon him against his father and setting an example for the younger siblings. Patricia affirmed that she "was always grateful that all you kids stood up for James."

James had been losing interest in school. His academic work continued to suffer even after coming out to his family. Mark recalled that "he started off very seriously as pre-med. He was encouraged by a lot of people because of his intelligence, but his heart wasn't in it. I think there were a lot of distractions being away from home. The freedom overwhelmed him." The Sakakuras had a distant cousin who was in medical school at

UC Irvine keeping tabs on James. That cousin confirmed that James "was not focused."

Soon, James dropped out of school. Like many gay men at the time when AIDS was just beginning to rear its ugly head, James continued to experiment with both drugs and sex. Neither Mark nor Patricia could pinpoint the moment when James became HIV positive. Mark remembered meeting Morrell, whom James introduced as "one of my good friends," when Mark visited James at a rehab residence. Mark said, "The first time I shook [Morrell's] hand, I looked into this person's eyes and said to myself, 'This isn't good.' I just got the shivers. In subsequent meetings, I felt the same way. I had met his other friends from the rehabilitation program, they were really nice." But Morrell had always given Mark an eerie feeling, and to this day, he suspected that Morrell had something to do with James's getting sick.

Morrell was James's boyfriend around that time. According to an essay collaboration among Joël Tan, Ric Parish, James, and James's lover Brian Green, published in 1996 (the year that James passed), Morell and James had a tumultuous relationship. So doomed was it that Brian had patiently waited, in what he called a "vigil" in the essay, for its demise so that he and James could be together.

Brian and James began dating in 1986. Brian was the third person to know that James was HIV positive. He was not deterred by James's revelation. James wrote in the essay, "Quiet and composed, he had stood up from the bed. . . . He paced back and forth a few times, then sat down, turned and hugged me. He said it didn't make any difference to him, that life was full of risks and that he was willing to become infected with HIV to be with me." In the same essay, Brian wrote, "It was never about sex. . . . Five years of making love went by before my tight-lipped kisses gave way to wet deep smooches. But baby, let me tell you I have never given myself so completely, fallen victim to the joy of him laying beneath me or on top of me, or gazing into eyes that love me." Brian tested positive for HIV in 1993, and they continued to be together until the very end.

But in the 1980s, James found himself in and out of rehab. Fortunately, he was waiting tables at a downtown restaurant that allowed him to go get help. Mark said, "Everybody liked him so much, and they kept him on so that he could have health insurance." Over the years, James racked up his problems with HIV, substance use, and codependence like bad debts. He fell ill once and had to be admitted to the San Pedro Peninsula Hospital. The providers there recommended that the family come together for counseling.

His family didn't hesitate. Outnumbered, even the father went along. While Mark conceded that his father by then had "toned down a lot because he knew how everybody felt," his patriarchal tendencies were still evident in these sessions. Patricia said, "I used to get so angry because they'd ask me a personal question, and my husband would answer for me. I said, 'I have a mouth of my own. I can speak for myself.' He wanted to be in control of everybody."

Shortly thereafter, Patricia realized that she couldn't live with her husband anymore. "So I divorced him," she said.

After her divorce, Patricia moved next door to her niece in a trailer park in Long Beach and began to spend more time with James, often chauffeuring her son to various medical appointments. These appointments piled up, and she found herself taking more and more time off from her job at Toyota. She remembered her employer being "very sympathetic." Even after she'd let them know why she needed the leaves, "they didn't question anything," she said. On these car rides to the doctor, she became reacquainted with her son. The whole family had to read up on AIDS and the available treatments. "I tried to find out what this whole thing was," said Mark. "There wasn't really a lot of information, and everything was experimental or the medications had terrible side effects." Once he learned more about HIV, Mark became an advocate. As a dentist, he started treating a lot of James's friends, including those who were HIV positive, on a sliding scale. "[Many dentists] didn't want to have anything to do with patients like that. I'd say, 'You guys are crazy. I kiss my brother. I'm not sick. You just do what you would for a regular person. You clean everything, anyway. HIV doesn't exist outside the body, like hepatitis.' It was just the ignorance. I was way past that."

Patricia said that James was hopeful about his survival: "He wouldn't have been taking the medication if he didn't think he was gonna get better. Initially, it helped." Mark added, "He definitely had hope. A lot of the support came from within the community, Brian and their friends. They rallied around him to keep the mood light and hopeful." Though Patricia

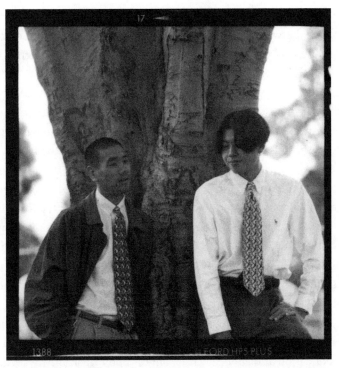

FIGURE 16.1. Former APAIT staff members James Sakakura and Dredge Kang. Courtesy of Robert Berger.

was open about her son's illness with her coworkers, she and the family couldn't find much solace in the local Japanese American community. James found the AIDS Intervention Team for support, and in the early 1990s, he became one of the outreach staff, working closely with Dredge Kang (figure 16.1). James forged such an intense bond with the people at the Asian Pacific AIDS Intervention Team (APAIT), especially the younger members of the staff at the time, like Joël Tan and Napoleon Lustre, that his family had even met some of them.

From working with other young activists at APAIT, James became "radicalized" and soon adopted the in-your-face attitude about his status and his activism. Joël recalled that "Napoleon had a thing about going to the swap meets because we aspired to be hood rats. That's how we defined masculinity in LA. [At a swap meet], James got this cap that had PWA [people with AIDS] embroidered on the front and Jap in the back. It was like a big 'fuck you' kind of thing to do. I still have his cap."

Dean Goishi said James "was excellent, from the very start. He was empathetic, he was always there, he did his outreach without complaining. And he was well-liked by staff." James was brazenly open not only about his HIV status, but also the fact that he was in recovery. "He never hid it," Dean said. "He tried to exhibit the example of someone who could live with the virus and be healthy and not dwell on the negative side of things. I think he was projecting himself as a very positive role model, that everything is not death and gloom." As he became the face of AIDS in the local Asian American community, James caught the attention of a public relations company in Japan, which had to look for an HIV-positive speaker of Japanese descent outside of their home country to come and speak to young people for their annual AIDS Day. Patricia accompanied James on this trip, flying into Osaka and being driven to Tokyo for the presentation. She said James was surprised to see how many young people came to hear him speak, and even more so when many of them came up to him after the presentation and asked questions.

"It was a huge moment for him," said Joël, "to represent as somebody who is in recovery and living with HIV." Back in LA, he doubled down on his education and advocacy role, but his body wasn't always willing to go along. James and Napoleon, another HIV-positive outreach staff member, often relied on Tylenol to make it through the workday. "Me and James had so much in common," Napoleon said. "We both went to UC Irvine and dropped out. He was six years older than me but we had the same birthday. We were both waiters at some point in our lives. Joël used to joke that James was like me, except he was sickly." While Napoleon could continue to show off his muscular arms in tank tops, James became skinnier and skinnier.

In 1996, Joël left APAIT and moved to San Francisco for a new job. Leaving James behind, as he got sicker, was very hard. The two shared an indelible bond. James first met Joël at one of his readings, at the end of which, James came up to Joël, "just sure and confident," and said, "We're just meeting but I think you're supposed to be my best friend." Joël must have sensed the same connection, for he replied, "I think you're right." James was by no means the first person with AIDS that Joël knew, though his friendship with James was the most "profound." Over the years, "burying" friends who succumbed to the epidemic led to many a sleepless night for Joël. He would experience what he called "lucid dreams"—a sort of out-of-body experience where he was conscious that it was out of sync with reality:

> James and I had regularly connected through these dreams. There was a dream that recurred several times where I woke up in my childhood home in the Philippines. Next to the home, outside of my living room window was a field where a carnival was setting up. And James was there. He took me by the hand and he pointed to the carnival and said, "That is what your life is, not this darkness." In another dream, I was washing his body in a tub and I was sensing from him that this was how I would usher him out. I remember waking up and James was there. I had such a hard time with insomnia that I could only sleep around James. I told him I had a dream, and he said, "I remember the bathtub. It's okay."

These psychic connections were so "natural" and intense that Joël wondered whether he and James were meant to be lovers, not just best friends. They even had discussions about it, but each time, they decided "it wasn't coming up for" either of them to be lovers. James told him, "We're supposed to be exactly who we are to each other."

Before Joël left for San Francisco, he told James, "Bitch, you're going to fucking call me if you're going to die, okay? I'm not kidding." A few weeks later, as he was just getting settled into his new job, he got that dreaded phone call. By then, James had stopped taking the medication, which was becoming much too potent for his weakened body. His mother said toward the end that James tried to talk but couldn't. His speech would slur, and he couldn't think straight. "I'm through with the medicine," he told his mother. Knowing the end was near, James asked Joël to come home.

"So I got on the plane in my usual style," Joël recounted. "I spent three days in his West Hollywood apartment. We rented videos. I rented *Beaches* and *Terms of Endearment*, and all those mother/daughter movies. We sat in bed and watched them. I got him a wig, too, and we ordered a shit ton of food. We spent those three days saying goodbye. He assured me that it was going to be okay. He said, 'Your life isn't going to be like this. Don't despair.' The next morning, he was gone."

Always armed with bravado, Joël broke down at this point of our interview. "[James] always told me to keep laughing, keep cooking, keep doing my thing. That it's okay to be an outsider and I'm not crazy. There were others I buried. He's just the one that I've had the hardest time letting go of. James knocked me out. I didn't know how to process it. No wonder I was so fucking angry."

Joël decided to process this grief the best way he knew how—through community building, by bringing people together to collectively mourn and celebrate James's life, by reading poetry, something that he and James had shared. For Joël, James reinforced the litany of death and legacy that fueled many AIDS activists:

> With all those folks that I buried, every single one of them expressed in some way, "We are now part of you. You carry on." To this day, when I have moments of ennui or depression, I remember all of the deathbed promises. And very clearly, I just snap out of it by thinking, "How dare I? How dare I waste a minute of my life indulging this when I'm carrying so many people with me who wanted to live, who wanted to experience middle age, who wanted to experience the dullness, the listlessness, the 'no ideas what to do'"? I agreed to carry them with me, so snap the fuck out of it, bitch, is what I tell myself. Snap the fuck out of it. You're not just living for you.

James's death shook the agency. Many among the staff had reeled from clients dying from AIDS, but it was the first AIDS-related death of a fellow staff member, especially one who was as well-liked as James. Noel Alumit, who had known James even before APAIT, said, "His death was really upsetting to all of us. We all loved him, and we all had crushes on him. I remember going to see his body and I was feeling really numb, just incredibly numb." Like Joël, Noel was trying to turn his grief and heartbreak into fuel for the AIDS work. He continued, "[James's death] was a really big wake-up call to a lot of us as far as why the work that we do is really, really important."

Noel remember Karen Kimura Joo breaking down at the funeral. Karen described his passing as both "devastating" and "pivotal." Both their families came from the South Bay. She said, "I knew his mother. His mother was like my mother. I knew how it affected the family. It just made everything so real and concrete, and it was difficult for everybody, including a lot of the clients. I almost thought, 'Can we survive this?'"

Even others on the periphery of the agency could feel the weight of their collective grief. Although Heng Foong couldn't tell me much about James, she had vivid memories of the time she sat with APAIT staff at his memorial and how they all cried. Naomi Kageyama saw how his death, the "first loss" of the agency, became a "turning point" for APAIT. "The unfairness of it really hit home," she said.

People grieved differently. There were those, like Joël, who were demonstrative. Dean, whom one staff described as a "father figure who had to stay strong," decided to commemorate James publicly by naming the clients' dayroom the James Sakakura Family Room. Dean said, "Somebody came up with the idea, which I thought was very good because that's where all the HIV-positive clients congregate." (APAIT has moved several times since then, but no matter the location, that room carries James's name.) Patricia spent a couple of months in this room making the AIDS quilt for her beloved son. The Japanese company that brought James to Japan contributed the clouds and Mount Fuji as the background, symbolizing his time in his ancestral homeland. Patricia added the rest: the years of his birth and passing, a photo of a healthy James with a relative, James's favorite cat, and a dolphin (something that James had hallucinated in one of his hospital stays). The quilt (block number 05216) went on display across the country with others. After his death, Patricia also went on a couple of AIDS Walk fundraisers with APAIT staff.

A few retreated. Eric Reyes appreciated these divergent ways of grieving. "Joël had a gathering to mourn," he said. "Back then, he just wanted to feel everything deeply all the time. I remember thinking maybe I should have gone, but I just couldn't go. It wasn't so much that I didn't feel for [James's] passing. There's something to be said about collective mourning, but that's just not my way. I wasn't the only one. [Joël] understood." For Napoleon, who had his own occasional struggles with T-cell counts, James's death hit much closer to home, and the grieving was much more private. "After James passed," he said, "Joël would be calling me, and James would be sending messages through Joël to come by. I just couldn't get it together to be present for him. The whole staff attended his funeral, and I was, I'm sure, just conspicuously absent. I couldn't be around people to see me in the mess that I was. Everybody left me alone about it. Nobody got in my face, nobody questioned it. Everybody knew

I was having a difficult time. And they respected it, the way we know how to do culturally." After thinking about it more, he added, "Maybe we're too good at it."

Even as a volunteer back then, I knew how devastating James's death was, not only to APAIT, but also to the local queer Asian community. I had shared a stage with him at a reading that Irene Suico Soriano organized for her *Wrestling Tigers* series at the Japanese American National Museum, and I had witnessed how under Irene's curation, James turned a very mainstream Asian American space into a queer one, even if for a night. I dreaded my interview with Patricia and Mark. Do I want to make a woman in her late eighties relive the trauma of her son's death and do so in front of her surviving eldest son? I thought I could offer in return the solace that James mattered to a whole lot of people; some, like me, he barely met. There was some of that; they were pleasantly surprised, for instance, that the family room at APAIT was still named after James, after two decades and a few relocations. But my dread was unwarranted. The two were as open as James would be about his struggles with AIDS and addiction. Perhaps this candor was another safekeeping of James's legacy. Mark had thought that in James's last days, they would spend more time looking back on their childhood, to the days when, he said, "we were still growing up. We're just brothers. I'm going to school. James is doing his poetry and writing and carrying on things that are important to him." Instead, they focused on forgiveness. "[James] said people who were hostile were searching for themselves and that you need to come from a place of love to understand and to accept someone who's either ill or has a different lifestyle. I think he was very forgiving towards others."

I asked Mark if he thought James had made peace with their father.

"I think so," he said. "From his end. And I think my dad eventually accepted his condition."

Patricia added, "He was always a gentle person. I was grateful that, Mark and the siblings, you were all close. I'm sure James was grateful that you all were there for him, too. That was important to me. I love you all for that."

CHAPTER 17

Not to Be Dicked Around

SALLY JUE WAS ONE OF THE EARLY FEMALE STAFFERS AT AIDS Project Los Angeles. One day, a coworker approached her and said, "I just wanted you to know that a bunch of us think the education director has the best body and you have the best legs." He mentioned a third winner, but Sally was so flabbergasted that all she heard was how he ended with a declaration: "It's pretty unanimous." Sally recalled another incident: "I couldn't believe that two gay men debated for twenty minutes the merits and the demerits of a dress I wore to work, while I was sitting there in the same office, instead of taking care of official business. It's absurd." She concluded, "Yeah, gay men can be just as sexist, and sometimes they think it's okay because they're not going to hit on you, or physically or sexually assault you." Some gay men might even write off that kind of "queer eye" commentary on fashion and appearances as some sort of gay sensibility. Many women had to "tolerate" these behaviors in a professional environment, which illustrates that a gay-male-dominated AIDS industry was still a male-dominated one and carried much of the baggage that came with it. "Some people get it when you bring it to their attention," Sally said. "Others take a little longer."

Women were the allies in the struggle against AIDS that every movement needs, a conduit through which people could slowly build sympathy toward a stigmatized population. Sally acknowledged that "women were less threatening." She elaborated: "We wouldn't necessarily tell people we were straight, [unless] I could leverage that to make people more comfortable. . . . In those situations, it was advantageous because people couldn't write me off as 'pushing an agenda.'"

Karen Kimura Joo similarly thought that the ethnic media she worked with to promote AIDS awareness were less guarded with her as a straight woman. She said, "At that time, HIV and AIDS was so stigmatized. When a woman was doing the work, it broke down some of those barriers. People were willing to listen and change their viewpoints." "I was straight," Naomi Kageyama added. "I was starting to become known as someone who could help bring in funds. I was a young professional who wasn't considered someone who would make waves—that's how I might have presented myself, or how people would view me. All those items made me more acceptable in most arenas. I'm just going to talk very candidly. In the provider network, I was more acceptable than, say, someone who was openly gay."

Dean credited the straight women he closely worked with, like Sally, Karen, and Naomi, with destigmatizing AIDS in the Asian American community. As Asian Pacific AIDS Intervention Team (APAIT) became more committed to working with immigrant communities, it was hard to find staff with the right language skills who were also LGBTQ *and* willing to be out in their communities. They often had to hire straight people, both men and women. Straight allies, particularly women, helped make that case that AIDS is not a gay disease. They helped ease the conundrum of the AIDS movement being a vehicle for LGBTQ leadership development while trying to tell the broader community that anybody could be at risk of becoming HIV positive (in other words, we wanted to own the movement, not the disease).

If women were allies to gay men in the AIDS epidemic, the relationship was not always reciprocal. After the Ryan White CARE Act was first passed, other US Department of Health and Human Services programs, like the Substance Abuse and Mental Health Services Administration, Office of Minority Health and Centers for Disease Prevention and Control, also began to invest in AIDS work, especially under the Clinton administration. The funding for AIDS treatment and services had leapfrogged those for women's health issues, like breast cancer. In her essay "New Alliances, Strange Bedfellows: Lesbians, Gay Men, and AIDS," Ruth L. Schwartz, poet and AIDS educator, wrote about the first lesbian AIDS caregivers conference in San Francisco in 1989. Schwartz recounted how Jackie Winnow, a lesbian involved in both AIDS and cancer work, challenged the audience to think about the disparity in public health resources between AIDS and breast cancer: "No one takes care of women or lesbians except women or lesbians, and we have a hard time taking care of ourselves, of finding ourselves worthy and important enough to pay attention to. . . . How is it that we are here today as lesbians working on AIDS?" Her question had two dimensions: the first, in Schwartz's words, asked "What *had* led us, community-minded lesbians, to such intimate involvement with an epidemic which appeared to affect so few of our own?"; the second asked where the gay men were in the fights for more prevention and treatment services for breast or ovarian cancer that afflicted the lesbian (and more generally, women's) community.[1]

One common explanation of women's allyship in the AIDS epidemic is that many of them were already socialized into helping professions, like nursing and social work. Sally was a perfect illustration of this. She had been a practicing social worker when she met her first AIDS patient, which altered the course of her career. Relationships and identifications with gay men also drew many queer women to the cause. As Schwartz explained, the early LGBTQ activism that predated AIDS "had forged alliances between some gay men and lesbians, setting the stage for cooperation in this new crisis. Lesbians in their twenties and early thirties living in San Francisco in the mid-1980s were more likely to know a gay man with HIV than a lesbian with cancer. . . . Many of us were also spurred by a broader sense of concern for, and political identification with, the larger gay community."[2]

That shared sense of "political identification" was how Unhei Kang became initiated in the AIDS movement. Teri Osato, a leader in Asian American queer women's organizing since the late 1980s, was a point of connection between APAIT and other women, including Connie Wong (who later became cochair of Los Angeles Asian Pacific Island Sisters [LAAPIS] with Unhei and an early member of the APAIT advisory board). Certified as a physical therapist in 1989, Connie had been working at the AIDS ward at County/USC. She said, "I remember all the precautions that we had to take. There were a lot of deaths on that ward." When Connie started dating Heng Foong in the early 1990s, Heng remembered that Connie had to get tested for HIV every six months because an incident with a patient might have exposed her to the virus.

The invisibility of gay Asian men in AIDS discourse and the injustices they suffered struck a chord in many queer women. Diep Tran also saw her AIDS activism as a broader transformation in sexual liberation:

> For me, the issues of AIDS and abortion are actually really close. Being raised in a Catholic family, you have to be anti-abortion. I was confirmed in high school, and we had to do community service. One of the community service was protesting outside an abortion clinic, carrying signs like Unborn Fetuses Discarded. Even then, I just couldn't square myself with that belief. I couldn't rebut the argument that you were killing something, but I couldn't, in good conscience, deny someone if they felt like they needed to have [an abortion]. I felt that it was wrong to make someone else do something just because you thought it was wrong. I understood, in some instinctive way, it was a civil rights issue.

Diep's feminist convictions were reinforced, she said, by "so many moments in my family when the women were just dicked around and the priest would just say, 'Give it to God. This is your burden to bear.' It was always the fucking women who had to bear the burden." She recalled an aunt who had planned on "getting her tubes tied" after yet another unplanned pregnancy. "The priest said, 'Oh, you can't do that. It's a contraceptive.' She couldn't use a condom, and she couldn't get her tubes tied. My uncle pretty much said, 'Okay, I won't touch you.' I just felt, 'What the fuck?' One, you have to rely on your husband to regulate this for you. Two, you're forced to be celibate." She saw the parallel in the sexual denial that was enforced in the gay community during the AIDS epidemic. To Diep, the AIDS movement wasn't just a health issue, but like the woman's right to have a safe abortion, it had broader implications on sexual freedom.

Many women also insisted that they were not at the periphery of the crisis; they championed women living with HIV who often were just an afterthought in the broader landscape of AIDS services and research. In that sense, describing the contributions of women in AIDS activism as allies (implicitly to gay men) may have the effect of minimizing the risk women had in contracting the virus, rendering them even more invisible. In the Asian American community, straight women who were living with HIV contracted the virus, often unknowingly, from their male partners who had engaged in sex with other men or were intravenous drug users. As the emotional support coordinator, Pauline Kamiyama organized the first support group for HIV-positive women at APAIT in 1994. "Many of them were angry because they didn't know their partners were having sex with men," she said. "Women also had their own issues with medications, because not enough clinical trials were done with women." That was the impetus of bringing them together in a space separate from the usually predominantly gay male support groups. In the beginning, there were only a handful of women, and most of them lived in Long Beach and Orange County, and the support groups were held offsite, away from APAIT's downtown office, at either someone's house or a restaurant. Pauline remembered a Vietnamese client named Jennifer who became an active spokesperson for APAIT: "Jennifer contracted it through heterosexual contact. She was young and open to sharing. She became the poster child for Asian women and AIDS."

It wasn't just straight women who were at risk. "Everyone is at risk," Unhei said, "because what you identify and who you have sex with could be two different things. We were focusing on women, including lesbians, and telling them that if they have ever had unprotected sex, they should get tested." There is a men's risk category called MSM (men who have sex with men) focused on the risk behavior rather than a self-avowed identity. Are some lesbians WSM? Yes, said Alice Y. Hom, who served on APAIT's community advisory board. She explained that "for lesbians, there was almost this idea of 'You don't have to worry [about HIV].' I do think women who were into S/M and having sex with men, probably gay men, should practice sex safely." Many sexual communities, as Alice and others referred to as "kink," did not adhere so strictly to these sexual identity categories. "How [AIDS] affected you is dependent on what kind of subcultures you were part of," she said.

Dean admitted that he was slow to hire women, especially for community outreach, which was the biggest unit at the agency in its inception years. He was aligning his programs with the prevalent funding categories that didn't include women. He said, "It came up at the community board why we didn't do more outreach to women and why we didn't hire more women. My answer was, 'Well, our target population is gay men, and our programs are highly geared towards gay men.' Therefore, the rationale was to hire gay men." More vexed by working limited resources to cover the diversity of the ethnic and linguistic communities, he thought it was "more urgent to hire people from multi-ethnic Asian communities than it was for gender."

Eric Reyes said, "It isn't necessarily that [Dean] didn't care about women. It's context and priorities. There was a documented risk and it wasn't just for representation's sake." Gay men were the primary target population, and Dean thought he needed to have gay Asian men on staff to reach and talk to their own. That was the conventional wisdom of "culturally competent" outreach that Dean thought he needed in order to secure funding for the infant organization. For the younger generation—people like Joël, Alice, and Unhei—the context was different. "[They] had the same priorities," Eric continued, "but understood that if you want to get at the underlying social justice issues which created this problem, you need to practice some kind of radical change, and that includes actually allocating resources to other communities which are not getting the resources simply because of their category." With the clamoring for women's programming, Dean knew he had to do something. To his credit, he recruited lesbians, such as Connie and Alice, to the advisory board.

When Alice joined that board, Dean told her, "We're really glad you're here. You're the first lesbian on the advisory board." Dean thought that with Alice's addition, APAIT could, Alice said, "start doing work or paying attention to Asian American lesbians and HIV education. He hadn't wanted to speak for Asian American lesbians, and he felt like he couldn't do anything until Asian American lesbians were there." Alice thought Dean was influenced by his experience at A/PLG, where the voices of its female members were often overwhelmed by men, especially White men. But she contended that there had to be a better way for co-gender organizing, because sometimes, deferring to women meant delaying resources to women, too.

"Men feel like they shouldn't talk for women," she said. "[That's a] good thing. What the men are saying, though, is 'So until we have a lesbian here, until we have a woman here, we're not gonna do anything.' As I think about it later, wow, that's just so fucked up because that would mean you're not gonna do anything about anybody until that person is here." To her, there might be many legitimate reasons why members of a marginalized group would take time to join a dominant group, even when the latter was well-intentioned. "What you could be thinking about," Alice continued, "is teaching yourself about the issues or how we could incorporate women with sensitivity."

These pitfalls in co-gender organizing in the AIDS movement were not unique to the Asian American community. In her study of ACT UP/ LA, Benita Roth found that the establishment of a Women's Caucus in that organization in 1990 sometimes offered a pass for the male leadership not to meaningfully address issues specific to women with AIDS. Similar to Alice's observations, Roth wrote, "Sexism was disguised as deference, and deference structurally sanctioned male ignorance of women's issues."[3]

In the mid-1990s, a community-based organization in the Vietnamese community in Orange County had received some HIV funding that required them to set up a community advisory board. Diep Tran, an APAIT staff member and a leader in Ô-Môi, a support group for queer Vietnamese women, remembered attending one of the first meetings for the board, where a homegrown gay male Vietnamese leader was selected as the chair. "You should have this be co-gender," she suggested. "There should be gender parity here." The men agreed but didn't know who they would nominate. Diep was getting impatient, and having been a student activist not too long ago, she knew sometimes you had to take matters into your own hands. Exasperated, she volunteered herself as cochair. "The fact that I was a woman sitting right in front of them saying that they should have gender parity, and they go, 'What? How can we do that?'—bitch, I'm right in front of you!—tells you a lot about that culture, and how it was so hard to break out of that," she reflected.

Dean heeded the voices from the younger generation, and in time, APAIT initiated one of the earliest HIV programs for Asian American women in the country. In 1992, APAIT established a women's action committee that would include both advisory board members, staff, and clients. They organized a support group for Asian American women with HIV. There was dedicated outreach to educate Asian American women about their HIV risks, including safer-sex workshops to lesbians and bisexual women at organizations like LAAPIS (figure 17.1). Staff like Unhei and Diep took their own initiative to build community for queer Asian women as part of the job description.

To Dean's happy surprise, women weren't just extra bodies; they made valuable contributions to outreach to gay men in substantive

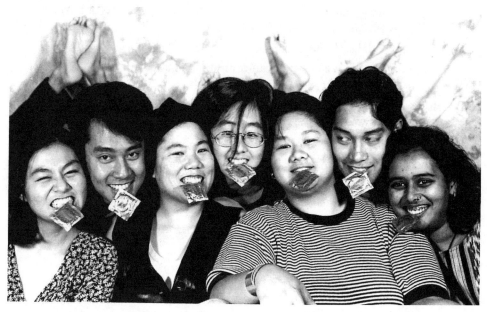

FIGURE 17.1. Image from Women and AIDS campaign. Courtesy of APAIT, a division of Special Service for Groups, Inc.

ways. In the early 1990s, the gay Asian community in LA was just coming out of this hegemonic period where gay Asian men were depending on mostly White men to enter the mainstream gay community, and where many gay Asian men did not approach people who looked like them for sexual, romantic, or even platonic relationships—the kind of racialized dynamic that early APAIT staff tried to disrupt with the Love Your Asian Body campaign. Because of internalized racism and homophobia, some gay Asian men actually found it easier to talk to women than other gay Asian men. As J Craig Fong explained, "I can imagine in some cases [gay Asian men] felt that this was a sister, and they could talk girl talk, and they could bond in a way that they didn't feel they could with another man."

Having women in the room inevitably changed the culture in the organization. Eric explained, "It wasn't like all the men, myself included, were sexist pigs when there were no women around. We're all sexist. What's important, though, is how you're articulating those biases in your behavior. . . . With Unhei in the room—and Unhei was pretty strong-willed—it forced us to act a certain way, even if it was just remembering consciously that it [AIDS work] wasn't just about the men."

Many of the men began to "broaden [their] consciousness" and learn how AIDS manifested differently for women and became strong advocates for their female clients. "The number one thing killing women with AIDS was their doctors," Ric explained. "It was their ignorance, and they didn't listen to women. All the research emphasis was on men, and specifically gay White men, because they were already in the system. Women were already getting diagnosed very late in the game because the symptoms were different, like pelvic inflammatory diseases and chronic yeast infections." And when they presented these symptoms that were not part of what was in the prevalent research, the medical profession dismissed them. Noel Alumit remembered Christine, an APAIT client who later joined the staff: "Her health kept deteriorating. And her doctors at the time kept saying, 'It's not AIDS related.'" Her death was quick and heartbreaking. Noel continued, "When Christine died, it was like, 'There's something wrong here.' She had a traditional Vietnamese funeral where people wore white. Christine was part of the women's committee, so people from that committee came to her funeral. It was really hard."

Women's programming did flourish at APAIT for a while. Most of the women's programming fell under the prevention arm of APAIT, which Dredge Kang oversaw. He recalled, "We had to do a lot of processing around women's programming in the agency, and we made certain kinds of commitments in terms of using discretionary funding." Without a dedicated funding source because the category "Asian American women" was not considered a priority for government funding, women's programming had depended on more fickle foundation funding and private fundraising. Despite these "commitments," however, in those years when funding became scarce, the women's program was also the first to be cut back or even eliminated. Tracy Nako remembered those "difficult" times: "We were on a momentum, and then all of a sudden we lost funding. It was like two steps forward and one step back." Dredge said that these were some of the "roughest patches" during his time at APAIT: "There's always this balance between what you can get money for and what the community wants. That balance was always a negotiation. There were lots of tearful meetings."

Sometimes, staff working on the women's programming would be transferred to another contract, and other times, they would be laid off. "The women's program always felt under siege," Diep said. While Diep understood that APAIT "mirrored the funding sources" and it was harder to raise funds to serve women than gay men, she felt that the agency could've tried harder. Some populations were just harder to reach because either they were not part of the funding priorities or the network or infrastructure in these communities was not as established. At least that was how the official line went. This applied not only to women, but also to the smaller ethnic communities. Diep said, "'They're harder to reach' was the excuse or the reason. If you're a Pacific Islander or Vietnamese, if you're a woman, it just gets boring and tiresome after a while."

Diep had been attracted to the radical beginnings of APAIT, and she got into AIDS work because she felt a sense of solidarity with her gay brethren. She recognized that she would hear about dicks and gay male sex more than most lesbians would care to. "I'm not a gay man," she said, "but for the same reason you get bashed, I get bashed, too. . . . So, to have spaces that were completely unabashedly validating to gay men and all their kink, to the principle of you can fuck whoever you want and not be bashed for it, was liberating for a dyke, too." She didn't mind that kind of gay male energy. What she couldn't tolerate was gay men "mansplaining women's orgasm" to her. Worse, supposedly co-gender community events showcased so little women-specific content that it was tokenizing to her. "These big events took up a lot of APAIT's time and energy," she said, "and the result was very gay male affirmative. If you're going to be gay men, then be all gay men. If you're going to take money and say it's co-gender, don't just pay lip service but fucking do a really good job of it."

In her recounting of ACT UP/LA's evolution, Roth found that in trying to advocate for women with HIV, women AIDS activists not only had to "make themselves visible to the heterosexist public and political establishment," but they also had to become visible to the gay male community, "to their fellow activists." Like ACT UP/LA, APAIT also operated under what Roth called "the problem of male epidemiological preeminence in the AIDS pandemic." In spite of this, women at APAIT were able to carve out spaces in a sometimes disagreeable environment for community building and leadership development that went broader than the AIDS cause.

Heng Foong had this recollection:

My office [PALS for Health] was across the hallway from APAIT, and one day, the women from APAIT were really upset about this letter that they had received from the Breast Cancer Early Detection Program. BCEDP was a statewide screening program that offered free mammograms for low-income women. They ran into my office with this letter that talked about the formation of an African American and a Latino task force, and there was no Asian Pacific Islander task force. It's the same thing—we don't register as data points. It's like, "Don't you think we exist?" We called BCEDP to get an answer. We wrote a letter. And eventually we met with them. I share that because it showed that these women were aware of the need within the community beyond HIV/AIDS. They were such strong advocates. That was one of the reasons why PALS began a women's health component.

For a long time after this episode, PALS consistently received funding from the local Susan G. Komen Foundation to provide interpretation and in-language promotion of breast health in the Asian American community.

The women's persistence in the AIDS movement allowed more opportunities for co-gender organizing in the 1990s than ever before. There were earnest intentions for men and women to be coconspirators in the movement. Yet missteps along the way had kept many women from feeling ownership of the movement.

In July 1993, just a year and a half after APAIT was formalized as a division of Special Service for Groups, Dean was able to get the National Minority AIDS Council to host its first ever API HIV/AIDS conference in Los Angeles. Called "A Question of Parity," the gathering of about 130 AIDS advocates and movement leaders was "a call to demand greater equity between the needs and resources of the Asian/Pacific Islander community." The goals included "to strengthen and promote collaboration between Asian/Pacific Islander AIDS agencies, service providers and advocates"; "to establish networks, share expertise and resources"; and "to lay a foundation for the development of a national Asian/Pacific Islander advocacy platform." Noel, who helped organize the conference, wasn't sure how APAIT was able to snag this honor. New York and San Francisco were considered the epicenters of the epidemic, and the infrastructure to address HIV/AIDS in the Asian American community were arguably stronger and more sophisticated in those cities. They had a longer history and more federal funding. Noel thought LA was appealing not only because of its Hollywood glamor—there was a handful of gay Asian men who were shot-callers in the entertainment industry—but also because of the city's variety of ethnic enclaves, which reflected a strong diversity of immigrant communities. He added, "I think part of it was that we all knew the most infected group was Filipino. Los Angeles had a big Filipino community that we could contribute to the conversation."

It was a big deal for the young organization. The keynote speaker included not only Michael Woo, the first Asian American on the LA City Council, but also Dr. David Ho, the famous AIDS researcher and early champion of antiretroviral therapy that led to better AIDS medications and dramatic reduction in AIDS mortality several years later. (In 1996, Dr. Ho was named Person of the Year by *Time* magazine for his breakthrough AIDS research.)

The night before the conference, the Gay Asian Pacific Support Network (GAPSN), a regular collaborator with APAIT, held a party for the conference goers at Circus Disco, a mega-gay bar in Hollywood. The event was meant to raise funds for local LGBTQ Asian American groups. Through a production company called Boy Toy, GAPSN organized a series of short performances for the night. One of the sketches, a parody, would pit men against women, and LA against everyone else.

Two Thai male performers—one in drag—were reenacting a scene from *What's Love Got to Do with It?*, the Tina Turner biopic that was released earlier that year. It was the scene where Ike Turner beats his wife, except the two performers were playing it campily for laughs. The audience, especially the women, were stunned. Sally Jue was there. She remembered that Fritz Friedman, an executive at Columbia/TriStar at the time who got the studio "to pony up some money" for the fundraiser, was the emcee for the event. Added to the offense of turning domestic violence into an extended punchline, one of the performers was also in blackface. "Everybody was horrified," Sally said. "Fritz did a good job with hustling [the performers] off the stage and moving things on." But the damage was done.

APAIT released a public statement the next day and offered "a brief description of what happened": "A group of women asked to make a statement re: racism (black face) and the abuse of women. . . . A self-identified co-chair of GAPSN responded as a supporting agency of the event, took the mic; and he said he respected the opinion of the women but he defended the performance content on the basis that it was entertainment and the intent was not to be offensive." The statement went on to "affirm the validity of the women's statements, [and] their right to speak out without being attacked." It continued, "APAIT as participant of the conference . . . accepts partial responsibility for not more carefully screening specific content of the performance. Last night reinforces the need for us to look at and deal with our own bigotry." The statement also acknowledged that "last night showed members of the API/lesbian/gay/ HIV communities still perpetuate sexist, racist, male dominant beliefs and actions, consciously and unconsciously."

The public statement, as well as most narrators in their interviews, recounted that one of the performers had been in blackface. However, at least one narrator disagreed with this characterization. "The Thai performers were dark skinned naturally," Dredge Kang said. "The person had a curly wig on, but there was no blackface, if I remember correctly." Having clocked many hours of field research in Thailand, he added, "In Thailand, they [imitate] Black performers with their natural skin color, and they just wear a curly wig, as opposed to actually putting on black makeup."

Ric Parish wasn't at the performance that night. He heard about the blackface the following day at the conference, but he, who is both Black and Filipino, was more forgiving even if that were true. He said, "If you're doing blackface, I should've been more offended than anybody, right? But I wasn't, because I know the context of who was doing it. I consider the source"—before he continued, I clarified that he was referring to the status of the Thai performers as presumably recent immigrants—"they didn't know better." Dredge described how an ideological tension around "what it means to be an English-speaking activist versus what it means to be like an immigrant working-class person" was simmering in these discussions. In this vein, those making a case about the "privilege" of the critics, he said, contended that their critique of the Thai performers was "classist."

I don't mean to derail a discussion about sexism in the movement with a detour into colorism, racism, and classism in the Asian American community. I do it to highlight how the incident almost immediately became *Rashomon*-like, with each witness telling a different version of the story based on their unique vantage point—during the conference, over the next twenty-four hours, and for months to come. Some of the organizers defended themselves by saying that as a volunteer-run organization, GAPSN didn't have the time and resources to vet every performance pulled together by the production company they hired, or they didn't think they had to because something like this had never happened before. As Ric argued, "Whoever booked them didn't know they were going to do that. It's not like 'Oh, you're going to do blackface and misogyny? Let's book them!' That didn't happen." Pleading ignorance or admitting to not having some due diligence didn't quell the critics, especially when emotions were running high.

Unhei recalled that the criticism that night, particularly made by women from Northern California, centered not only on the fact that the performance made light of violence against women, but also that it was done by a man in drag, when there was so little involvement of women in the entire production. Unhei was sympathetic to the first criticism, but less to the second. "It was complicated. There were so many layers. The performance wasn't sensitive to violence against women, I agree. But I don't think they were fair to the drag community, the transgender performers. They are also part of our community. They should perform." Her attempt to "pacify or placate the very angry and hurt women" was futile. Instead, the criticism turned on her as an APAIT staff member and a LAAPIS leader, which had cosponsored the fundraiser. "They felt we should have been stronger and stood up for it," she said. "I was getting scolded. I was chided even before I had any time to process what happened. There was just too much anger at that time."

Making matters worse, an altercation broke out in the parking lot between the women activists from out of town and Peter Corpus (likely the "self-identified co-chair of GAPSN" mentioned in APAIT's public statement). Some of the women allegedly felt physically threatened by him. The more the LA organizers defended themselves, the more these women felt dismissed and unheard. Alice, who was on the APAIT advisory board and also had close friendships with some of these women, remembered the whole incident as being "fucked up" to begin with, but it was made even more awful by the men (mostly) digging in their heels. She remembered thinking, "Fuck Asian American gay men for cheering it on saying that nothing was wrong with it, or saying it's just an act, cosigning with 'It's okay because it's a drag performance.' Once again, if the women weren't there [to call out the misogyny], it would've been fine, right? Do you want women to be a part of your movement or not? And if so, then you're gonna have to change how you do things."

Dean knew that the controversy wouldn't blow over by the conference next day. Early that morning, before the first panel, he facilitated a "strategy meeting" with the conference organizers, including Sally. She said, "We knew there was going to be blowback. We couldn't just pretend it didn't happen because there were a lot of people who were really upset about it, especially the women." The organizers quickly drafted the public statement that morning.

On behalf of APAIT, Dean made a public apology at the opening of the conference. Connie said, "There was a lot of outrage among the women involved in APAIT and LAAPIS. . . . I don't recall if the men were equally outraged, but I do remember Dean being very sad and apologetic, and on the verge of tears about it. . . . He said, we are on the big stage now. It was so personally painful to him to have to deal with this. He wanted to make sure APAIT did right by everyone, including the women in the organization, and he was very apologetic. Everybody agreed that we needed to support Dean." Noel remembered that "Dean got in front of everybody, and the staff and board stood behind him. That was also the very first time I saw Dean cry." Ric recalled that "a couple of lesbians stormed the stage" to express their grievances. Afterward, someone—Ric couldn't remember who, though he thought it could have been Paul Kawata, the director from the National Minority AIDS Council, which provided funding for the conference—tried to placate them and said, "Thank you for educating us, ladies." "Ladies!" Ric exclaimed. "That's a whole another narrative right there. That was like throwing water on a grease fire."

When it became apparent that a public apology would not give them the closure they needed to move forward with the conference, the organizers decided to set aside time to process what had happened the night before instead of the scheduled panel. According to Sally, "We made space to talk about what happened because it wasn't such a huge conference. All the women went to one room to hash things out and express themselves, and all the men went into another room to do that."

In the women's group, things escalated quickly. Sally was listening to what people were sharing. "Then," she said, "all of a sudden, one of the lesbians from San Francisco pointed at me and said, 'Why didn't you do anything?' I said, 'What do you mean?' And she said, 'When you saw what was going on, why didn't you get up and go stop them?' Somebody else piled on, and next thing I knew, there were three or four angry young lesbians blowing up at me. 'You live here. You know these people. You work with these people. You should've gone up and interrupted the performance.'" Without any of the men around, Sally became the "target"—similar to what happened to Unhei at the venue the night before. "I just got really pissed on. I let them go on for a while." When that kept going, she told her dissenters, "Look. You have no right to be calling me out. You are making all sorts of assumptions about my relationships with this group of people, much less the individuals involved with the performance." The reality was, Sally worked closely with people at APAIT, but she didn't have much relationship with GAPSN leaders, and none at all with the performers. While she was horrified by what the performers did, she, like Ric, understood (or assumed) that the performers didn't have the political and historical contexts to grasp how offensive their performance was. She said, "There is no way I would even dream of doing what the women were saying and create a big scene in front of all these people, and publicly embarrass them even more. We live with these people. We're going to have to deal with the fallout."

Sally stood her ground and fumed:

And I got up at seven in the morning with a bunch of other people, including Dean, so that we could decide how we were going to handle this. Collectively, at the conference and long-term. Do you have any idea what it's taken to even get to this place? We're not about to blow up all the relationships we have worked so hard for so many years to create, to even get to a place where people from Los Angeles will be willing to come out and participate in something like this. You're just going to come to the conference and go home and probably would never see most of these people again.

With that, she got up and left.

The conversation on the men's side went a little differently. "We did our own little workout," Ric said. While everyone in the group agreed that what happened was important to discuss and unpack, many, especially those who were HIV positive, were "feeling hijacked," according to Ric. Many had come to the conference for the rare opportunity of connecting with other Asian American AIDS activists from across the country. Now that energy was deflated underneath the "grumbling." Noel said, "There was some resentment in the room that all of a sudden, the focus from AIDS and HIV shifted to gender dynamics in an AIDS organization. Still really important, but what happens to this other very important discussion of AIDS?" Ric agreed: "I think it was important to address it [sexism], but I think it got too much attention—more attention than it needed to get. Not to marginalize my lesbian sisters of color who brought that to our attention, but you know, there's got to be a balance."

About a week later, GAPSN issued its own statement. It didn't help. The statement read, "GAPSN was not responsible for the Boy Toy performance or its content. The performance and benefit dance were not GAPSN function, but rather were organized by the Asian-American Alliance Against AIDS. However, because of the views publicly stated by some GAPSN members, many may believe their views represent GAPSN's views. They do not." The statement acknowledged that the performance was "insensitive" and "inappropriate to the purpose of the evening's benefit dance"; but the condemnations, if one could hear through the passionate ears of the critics, seemed mild. While admitting that racism and sexism were at play, qualifying the performance's "inappropriateness" implicitly suggested that there might be legitimate "purposes" where the act would be considered appropriate, and that this was just a lapse in judgment. The organization also threw its members under the bus by refusing to claim responsibility for it. (The underlining emphasis on "not"—twice—was not mine.)

Predictably, the activists from Northern California were not placated by this response and wrote a rebuttal to GAPSN. Because of Alice's relationships with these activists—she had worked in San Francisco briefly, after she came out as a lesbian and before returning home to LA—Alice was asked to cosign the letter. I don't have the final version of this letter, but Alice shared with me a draft dated August 19, 1993—it was faxed to her several days later—where she made suggested edits as requested by the collective of activists. Unlike the GAPSN letter that made vague references to offending "GAPSN members," this letter called out Peter Corpus specifically and his "response to the women's protest of this assault under the guise of entertainment against African Americans and women." The letter continued: "Mr. Corpus publicly dismissed and attempted to silence the women and their actions. He rallied the crowd of predominantly gay Asian Pacific Islander men against the women and their actions. Furthermore, he attempted to physically attack a woman during the aftermath of the incident." (Alice suggested replacing the last sentence with "He acted in a physically aggressive and threatening manner to a woman, so much so that individuals intervened between the two.")

Then, the activists from Northern California asserted that GAPSN was responsible because Corpus was its cochair. Citing GAPSN's own stated commitment in its letter "to educating its own members . . . about the necessity to take a stand against racism and all forms of individual and institutionalized violence against women and against APIs," these activists called GAPSN's bluff and challenged the organization to "remove Mr. Corpus as GAPSN co-chair." The draft was undersigned by a "partial list" of eleven activists, most of whom were women. One of the few men I noted on this list was Leo Y. Joslin, a former GAPSN member who now resides in the Bay Area. In the margin, Alice, ever the strategist, suggested adding more men to the list.

In the end, there wasn't much reconciliation after these letters were exchanged. Stuck in the middle between activists in LA and elsewhere, Alice now could reflect, "This event can't destroy these organizations. I don't think it was at that level." People wanted to be heard, and soon, much of this faded into memory. Sally said that one of the women who had taken her to task later called and apologized for the group. She accepted the apology, recognizing that emotions were running high in the immediate aftermath.

The event wasn't without repercussions. "People felt devastated," Dredge recalled. "I think a lot of people were super bitter. [The controversy] reinforced a lot of people's anxieties that LA wasn't like San Francisco or New York, because the critique came from outside, that we were not as progressive as these other places. It was a huge blow." There wouldn't be another "national API HIV/AIDS conference" for a long while. Locally, the brouhaha became something of a folk legend. JJ Joo, who wasn't working at APAIT then, had heard about it. His takeaway was that "maybe even the gay community hasn't gone far enough to be sensitive towards women's issues." Heng Foong, who had just moved to LA from Boston, remembered that the retelling of it in the queer Asian women's community "triggered some uneasy feelings" toward some of the gay male leaders.

Even within GAPSN, the controversy split the organization. A newer generation of leaders disagreed with how the older guards handled the situation. Jeff Kim, the chair of GAPSN's membership committee at the time, lamented how the event undid a lot of goodwill from the previous years of co-gender organizing, particularly with LAAPIS. Jeff became GAPSN's cochair the following year. He recalled having to repair these relationships. That new group of leaders did this partly by ushering in a more progressive and inclusive agenda, like promoting immigrant rights and supporting smaller ethnic-specific social groups.

Diep Tran was still a college student at UC Riverside when all this took place. When she joined the APAIT staff more than a year later, the agency was still "in the shadow of that kerfuffle." "In some ways," she said, "they were just a bunch of guys, albeit gay guys hanging out and being as misogynist as they wanted to be. When women called them out, they were like, 'You know what we mean' kind of attitude. All of a sudden now, they had to watch it a little more. The men were feeling a little touchy. It came up in conversation, like 'We don't need another Ike Turner.'"

There are many ways to tell a story, and I have struggled to find the best way to tell this one. It didn't help that while the memory provoked such strong reactions from the narrators, the actual recall of the events was scant or impressionistic. There were also missing viewpoints: the women activists from out of town, the Thai performers, and Peter Corpus, the center of so much ire. (Peter passed away in 2010.) In all accounts, the criticism of his reactions seems fair. What is not fair to Corpus is my retelling of this incident after his death, when his reflection, or perhaps even reconciliation, of what happened couldn't be recorded. And the retelling, in the context of AIDS movement history, isolated him from his contributions to the local gay Asian men's and Filipino American community, where he had been a backbone to more than one community organization. Like *Rashomon,* there is no easy way to tell this story completely and do justice to all involved.

Despite the event's many imperfections, I was always unwavering in my decision to include it as part of the movement history. To document only those stories of our community in which everyone got along would be neither true nor respectful; our community was never monolithic. This example alone showed the multiple positionalities—not only between men and women—that made the incident both so interesting and instructive. Like JJ, I heard about the event secondhand, and I had always assumed that the only progressive and feminist interpretation was the condemnation of the performance. It didn't occur to me until I talked to Sally and Unhei that the local women were put in the position of having to balance their outrage and their working relationships with these male-dominated organizations. From Ric and Noel, I learned that people living with HIV felt marginalized in the narrative and at a conference that was meant to grow their networking. And what of the Thai performers? If we believe the assumption that they, as recent immigrants, didn't understand why domestic violence was not comical or blackface was hurtful, no one sought their side of the story or tried to have a conversation with them as part of restorative justice. So little was known of them, in fact, that there was disagreement over whether one of them was transgender or in drag, or whether the other was in blackface or just dark skinned. Even in the three public statements that were released after the incident, the two performers were merely part of the facts, not people who needed to be part of the reconciliation.

The AIDS movement offered a rare co-gender organizing space for queer men and women in LA, not only through the hiring practices at APAIT, but also through supporting membership organizations like GAPSN and LAAPIS, who would in turn work together to sponsor

AIDS fundraising and education events. These relationships were probably why the local activists didn't react as indignantly as outsiders wished they had to the offending event. This left the activists from out of town so befuddled that they turned their wrath on the local women. These women, and those who came after them, didn't let this early setback deter them from leveraging this radical (if imperfect) space to build the queer Asian women's community that they collectively envisioned. But as the AIDS industry became more professionalized, that radical window began to close.

CHAPTER 18

Downright Respectable

IN THE EARLY 1990S, THE ASIAN PACIFIC AIDS INTERVENTION Team (APAIT) was just a scrappy agency scratching the door of the burgeoning AIDS bureaucracy in LA County. "We had very few Asians that had HIV experience or even social work experience," Dean Goishi recalled. "We were looking for a warm body that could be trainable into the functions that we needed that body for. They could learn on the job. We were looking for people who knew the community and who was passionate or enthusiastic. These were the critical ingredients to sustain the work. If they didn't have them, they'd burn out quickly. HIV/AIDS wasn't a nice environment to work in. If they were in it for the money, they would not last very long." Dean's "critical ingredients" were what the young activists had in spades. While basic hard technical skills, like organizing and case management, didn't hurt, Unhei Kang believed similarly that it was "being a bi woman, being ostracized by my family for my sexuality, [that] helped me to empathize and want to provide support" to people in her community.

The younger generation would add political analysis with a racial equity lens to this short list of qualifications. The other two cofounders, Joël Barraquiel Tan and Ric Parish, had been organizing with other radical queer people of color prior to APAIT and, in the post-AB101 climate (see chapter 4), had settled on AIDS as their battlefront to challenge the increasingly regressive culture around sexual liberation. Early staff were all self-starters interested in not just fighting the epidemic, but also using AIDS as a vehicle for community building and broader queer organizing. This political orientation drove the radical vision of APAIT in those years, attracting young queer Asians and making it *the* training ground for them. That APAIT was the biggest employer of openly LGBTQ Asian Americans in LA was one of Dean's sources of pride.

And these activists were definitely not doing it for the money, although the paycheck did provide some financial regularity (if not stability) for many early staff who were also writers, artists, and actors. Since most of APAIT's early funding was for outreach and education and most of the outreach happened in the evenings and weekends, the flexibility in work schedules left ample time for staff to practice their craft or go to auditions during the day. The job accommodated their artistic calling. In return, their talents were an asset to the fledgling movement. As Noel Alumit recalled, "That very first group, a lot of us were creative people. There was a big creative vibe to it." The staff came up with provocative ways to engage a community that didn't always want to have a conversation about AIDS. Even before the age of the internet and social media, technological advances had made graphic design, photography, film, and video-making more democratic, affordable, and accessible. With a small budget, APAIT was able to mount many social marketing campaigns.

Exemplifying the DIY spirit of independent arts production, young queer Asian writers and poets, through APAIT, were organizing themselves in writing circles, publishing their own literary journals and zines, and carving out spaces for poetry readings. These were all creative community building strategies for HIV prevention. A few APAIT staff members broke through and found success and recognition for their writing in the new millennium. Noel Alumit (*Letters to Montgomery Clift*) and Ghalib Shiraz Dhalla (*Ode to Lata*) began their debut novels while working at APAIT. They were both published in 2002. Joël Tan released a book of poetry, *Monster*, in that same year and went on to edit a series of queer erotica. All of them traced their inspiration to their involvement in the AIDS movement.

While these staff members brought much creativity to the budding agency, their office and administrative skills were less abundant. Public contracts require considerable paperwork and bureaucratic know-how. While APAIT staff members were surefooted in finding and talking with Asian MSM on the street, many dragged their feet with the tallying and the reporting of their outreach results back at the office. Even the most passionate writers among them balked at these assignments. Dean knew that his staff was doing good and impactful work, work that no other agencies in LA could do, but he would say that if they couldn't report the work to their funder thoroughly and correctly, it would be as if the work had not been done at all. He knew that for the agency to grow, it had to demonstrate that it could successfully navigate the arduous government bureaucracy.

The young staff also needed some direction. Noel said, "One of the reasons we were hired is because it was assumed that we would know how to talk to other Asian Americans, that they would be willing to talk to us more because we looked like them. We call it cultural capital now. There was some training on how to do outreach. We got all the AIDS 101s. But a lot of what we did was just hit and miss." Noel had to rely on his training in acting and marketing experience from East West Players to figure out the best way to approach and talk to other queer Asian men. Other staff members who entered the agency from different paths also brought their unique knowledge base to the work, but there was little space to synthesize and standardize. Even Joël, the self-proclaimed enfant terrible, acknowledged that the agency needed some structure. "You can't rule from a fighting horse," he reflected. "You've got to know when to battle and when to just take care of your kingdom. A lot of it was gut. We didn't know what the fuck we were doing, but we were following an impulse. None of us knew how to set up offices."

As J Craig Fong said, if a bit tongue-in-cheek to make a point, "Nobody enjoys grant writing. Nobody enjoys budgeting. Nobody enjoys personnel. It's no fun, but somebody's gotta step up and do that. Somebody's gotta take all the meetings and apply for all the funds so the rest of them can go and do the fun work. Holding hands, doing community organizing."

Staff meeting minutes from 1994 confirm increasing "growth management" concerns among staff, who often pressed for more "direction and structure, but with a vision." They wanted guidance on volunteer management, public relations, client intake, professional development, salary schedule, performance evaluation, and conflict resolution. Even dress code. After a staff member showed up to an HIV planning council meeting inappropriately, they had a discussion about it for at least two meetings. In the second one, Joël felt that "the use of common sense as our only guideline was inadequate." The team decided that for public meetings, staff should wear "a nice shirt or sweater and nice jeans or slacks. Consider jackets and ties if testifying."

Knowing he needed to bring in some help to professionalize the agency, Dean turned to Eric Reyes, whose academic training he valued. Eric was one of the young people whom Colors United brought to APAIT when it was still part of Asian/Pacific Lesbians and Gays (A/PLG). At that time, Eric had just started a master's program in urban planning at UCLA. Dean had already tapped Eric's talents, when he was spearheading the Asian Pacific AIDS Education Project. "Dean knew I was a student," Eric said. "He just thought, 'Oh he's smart. He can write.'" So confident had Dean been in Eric that he recruited—"more or less pushed," in Dean's words—Eric to replace him at the AIDS Education Project when he was making that transition to APAIT in 1992. When Dean began to think about managing APAIT's growth a few years later, he contracted Eric as a management consultant.

Eric wrote proposals for APAIT because he had a strategic mind for program design and knew how to gather research to support it. He said, "There's that whole scientific language around behavioral modification. Basically it's 'How do you get people to change their idea of what's right and wrong and how do they change behaviors according to that?' It wasn't my training, but in those days, those scientists didn't know that much either." Eric did have the critical thinking and writing skills to adapt whatever APAIT was doing in outreach and education and align it with what the academic literature was promoting in HIV prevention.

Eric also started to develop systems and protocols (finally), a structure for what had been a very loose culture at the agency. He wrote the personnel manual for staff and another for the advisory board in formation, developed tools for program management and budgeting, and designed programs. He knew his program design would work only if it was generated from the experience of the line staff, who also needed a sounding board for their ideas in a way that Dean didn't have the bandwidth or the expertise to provide. "A lot of what I did was helping people do their jobs, whatever that took," Eric said. "They needed someone to talk to who was not their direct report. That gave me a really good understanding of what people were doing and what they needed. So when I wrote a proposal, the program design would reflect that." As director, Dean also needed a trusted ear. Eric became a sort of ombudsman. "I talked to Dean pretty extensively," Eric remembered. "I know it was valuable for Dean to be able to talk to someone in a way that he couldn't talk to other people, because I was learned and thoughtful." Eric was beginning to leave an imprint on the organization in a way that made him think Dean was "grooming [him] to be his successor." He said, "I was pretty much managing everything internally and [Dean] was doing all the external work." Eric thought that might have led to some under-lying tensions between him and Joël at the time, "like who's the favorite son." He said, "Everyone was unconsciously manifesting daddy issues."

Looking back, Eric thought the middleman role he occupied at the agency capitalized on his strength: "It made me understand that I'm much better at being second. Much better at doing the nuts and bolts. Even though I can see the big picture, I'm not very good at articulating that and advocating that." He thought both Dean and Joël were two contrasting models of advocacy, the former relying on a respectability politics and the latter playing the part of agitational outsider. Despite their generational and stylistic differences, Eric thought the two "were so effective together: You don't want to talk to me? You get to talk to the other guy."

The increase in public funding was responsible for the explosion of staff, beyond just outreach and prevention to include case management, treatment advocacy, and even clinical services. In just a few years, its staff size had grown to close to twenty. It wasn't just the size of the staff that made the agency more complicated, but also the fact that some staff members had more "professional" training, like social work. AIDS had been developing into an industry, and APAIT was beginning to catch up with bigger and mainstream AIDS service organizations. The depen-dence on public dollars for AIDS services—something that the activists had been agitating for—also meant the agency would have to become more sophisticated structurally. Activism and professionalization were two ends of a see-saw that required diligent balancing, but the latter was weighing much heavier on one end with each staff person hired. By 1994, staff was expressing concern about overreliance on public funding, which accounted for over 90 percent of APAIT's budget. They wanted to diver-sify APAIT's income portfolio and increase foundation and private fund-ing so that they could be as nimble and creative as they had been at the inception of the agency—when they were less cumbered by the bureaucracy and the narrow parameters of public funding guidelines—without shrinking the staff size that the more restrictive public funding had made possible.

In the midst of this expansion, Dean realized that he couldn't manage all the staff and still work with the increasingly complex AIDS bureaucracy: "A good portion of my time was spent on the agency's development and advocacy. I was going to a lot of meetings—county, state, and federal." There were more and more meetings to attend and speak up at, so that APAIT wouldn't be "out of sight, out of mind" with policymakers. When invited, Dean jumped on and got involved with committees and advisory boards for these policy bodies to elevate APAIT's standing. Dean said, "Even if it didn't directly involve funding for APAIT, [the networking] let people know that our grants were actually legitimate and truthful, and we would do what we said we were going to do, and we would do a good job. I think they'd give us the benefit of the doubt before somebody else who might not have been involved [as he had been]." With funding success came more and more reports, documentation, audits, and renewal applications. Dean needed more than just systems and protocols to "set up offices."

As Dredge Kang explained, "When I started, we were basically a wheel-and-spoke model. There was Dean [at the center], and everybody else more or less reported directly to Dean. We met every week one-on-one with Dean and talked about what was going on with the programs. Once we started expanding, that was no longer possible."

As part of restructuring, Dean created a layer of middle management from three trusted members of his staff. He tapped Tracy Nako to develop a client services division, Karen Kimura Joo to oversee the community development division that worked with all the media and ran the social marketing campaigns, and a young Dredge to head the prevention division, which encompassed the largest number of staff at the time. Dredge said, "Then it became this pyramid structure with Dean at the top, the three of us reporting to him, and then each of us with programs that we ran." The changes were apparent not just in the organizational chart. "Working styles changed a lot," Dredge added. "Expectations changed a lot." Immediately, he put forth a different vision of organizing the outreach work. Until then, outreach staff were divided by funding sources, which had created some duplication, confusion, and even competition among staff members. In the 1995 board retreat, Dredge explained his plan of program integration this way: "Rather than state MSM outreach, county MSM outreach, city MSM outreach, we now have PSE [public sex environments] outreach, community outreach, monolingual outreach. Integration by program rather than contract allows staff to provide services in teams. Staff are able to support each other, boost morale, and increase safety; thereby providing more effective and efficient services."

The three divisions had to work more intentionally to coordinate. "We would still try to have interdepartmental communications to see how we could cross over and make sure that clients were being served in every possible way," Karen explained. "For example, we would give the fortune cookies [with prevention messages inside]. I totally relied on the outreach team to help write the prevention messages about HIV testing and HIV education because I was just one person."

With the new hierarchy, a lot of the administration Dean used to oversee was spread and shared with the new managers. When he was promoted to manage client services, Tracy recalled, "I was still doing case management at the same time, so I was doing two jobs. I was dealing with budget and hiring. I started being more involved with the board, just helping Dean whenever he needed something." Dean said, "It was not necessary for me to stay on top of them and look over their shoulders because they knew [their respective area] better than I did. If there was any conflict with a staff member, they would try to resolve it before they brought it to me."

The new structure might have made Dean's life more manageable, but his picks stirred the pot for the rank and file. Dredge described it as "a very difficult transition. It's also that period where there was this tension between the old guard and the new guard." There were others in the organization who had more seniority than the managers, including the other two cofounders, Joël and Ric. It also didn't help that the three people Dean chose were of East Asian descent (Japanese and Korean) in an organization that was fighting an epidemic that was hurting Filipinos disproportionately. And as passionate as the three were in AIDS activism, none was HIV positive. Dredge's selection perhaps created the most strain. Dredge was the youngest of the three and had dropped out of college to work for APAIT. Even then, Ric had seen Dredge as "academic"—the kind of "brain power" the agency needed to complement the activists. The cofounders had obviously seen enough signs of a wunderkind in Dredge, both through his passion and smarts, to recruit him from the East Coast. "They had first hired me as the program supervisor," Dredge said. "I came in one step higher than James [Sakakura]. . . . James was fifteen years older than I was, but I was his supervisor. Then as we grew, I was the one that was promoted." He acknowledged other staff who "thought they should've gotten my position because they had been there longer." As he quickly ascended another notch in the supervisory ladder, "those tensions only got stronger."

Some recognized that Dean was looking for specific skillsets in picking these managers. He needed people who knew how to comply with the bureaucratic requirements that would keep the agency financially afloat, people who could keep good financial records and program notes and who understood the systematic (but often convoluted) thinking of government funders enough to translate what was happening on the ground in technical terms that the bureaucrats could easily discern and accept. Tracy said his new position "allowed me to tap into my business education more." To those who didn't have a passion for the business side of things, these tasks just seemed like "pencil pushing."

Dean also didn't involve other staff members in making the decision; it came as a surprise to some. The tension was muted but unequivocal; Napoleon described it as a "quiet bitching and grumbling." A few people I interviewed spoke openly about their displeasure. One said the appointments were "such an insult in our face after we had innovated everything." The first-person plural referred to both Filipino staff at APAIT as well as the early staff who used their creativity and radicalism to reach out, educate, and build community. (When I first broached the subject with him, he half-jokingly asked whether I was trying to "lure him into a dangerous conversation about yellow colorism.")

Ric was disappointed by Dean's decision, though he understood why Dean made it. Ric, ever candid and measured, explained it this way:

> I think it was more who had degrees. I had those skillsets, but I'm a
> [college] dropout. Let me just say this. Dean Goishi was a pillar of
> APAIT. He was the reluctant leader. Joël and I knew that there's no
> way in hell that we could do it without him, but we also knew that he
> couldn't do it without us. Dean was fairly focused on the

infrastructure. We were the advocates who no longer asked politely. That was new. Joël and I—me half Black, half Filipino; Joël, this big Filipino guy that looks more Samoan—just scared the hell out of everybody. That's what happened. We needed each other's balance. We were all necessary because we were three legs of a tripod that could not stand without. Each one of us brought something. Ultimately, he was the leader and he had to make the tough decisions. I didn't always agree with all of his decisions, right, and some of his decisions infuriated me. But I had to keep my eye on the bigger picture. The bigger picture was we were making an incredible impact on the community. So these minor internal office politics were really irrelevant.

Not long after this restructuring, Joël left for a management position at another AIDS service organization. When he left that job to move to the Bay Area, that organization offered his position to Ric, which he left APAIT to take. With a $10,000 bump in salary, Ric finally got the promotion that he never had at APAIT.

Ric never thought that Dean's restructuring decision had to do with yellow colorism. He said, "The yellow/brown dynamic is rooted in the model minority myth, right? Brown Asians are the ones who are like the second-class citizens." As someone who is proudly Black and Filipino— he called it a "double indemnity"—Ric had lived a life "trying to navigate around that [model minority myth] and prove that I'm Asian, that I have the right to even speak on behalf of this population. I saw [colorism] in working with other API organizations, especially non-queer-centered organizations. I didn't see it within APAIT."

While I agree with Ric and others that Dean's decision might not be a direct product of yellow racism—even the one person who said it was an "insult" thought Dean "probably didn't have a clue about it"—I wouldn't go as far to say, as Ric did, that APAIT was immune from this bias. At least one person who had left the organization because of it didn't want to be interviewed for this project when I approached him. Most narrators, including Dean, indicated that Dean had a single-minded focus on infrastructure—it fell on his shoulders to keep the young agency afloat. He picked Tracy, Karen, and Dredge as an extension of himself in order to grow the organization. He might have used having a college degree (though Dredge didn't have one at the time, he clearly had an "academic" mindset) or palatability as an agency leader (over radicalism) as a criterion, but access to higher education and decorum, the early signs of professionalism, could be unconscious bases for the model minority bias. But at that point of the AIDS epidemic in the early 1990s, to survive was to professionalize. Dredge said:

> I don't think the activism left, but the tone was different than in the earlier days, when pride marches and protests were considered a large part of the work. As time went on, the work became more regimented. We had to do X number of this and Y number of that. That was not just us. The entire AIDS industry was professionalizing. If you look at the original APAIT crew, a lot of us didn't have degrees. By the time I left APAIT, people would expect somebody in my position to have an MPH. You'd expect people in direct services to have MSW or LCSW. And the [organizations] that died very early were the ones that did not professionalize at all. Those organizations were obliterated.

Another agency that survived and thrived was Bienestar. In the early 1990s, Oscar de la O, its founding director, was ruminating over his jump from activist to professional. Now with a multi-million-dollar budget serving the Latino community across Southern California, Bienestar, like APAIT, had a humble beginning as a volunteer committee at a membership-based LGBTQ organization in LA. With the infusion of AIDS funding, the committee quickly outgrew its parent organization, whose leadership, like A/PLG's, was somewhat indifferent to the cause. When Bienestar got its first county contract, Oscar allocated the entire budget to the health educators, while he continued to volunteer his time as the program's administrator. "I had my regular job [a manager at an accounting office]," he said, "and when I would get out at 4, I would come over to Bienestar and be there until 9."

The 1990 Ryan White CARE Act, the first substantial investment by the federal government to fight the epidemic, upended all that. Oscar explained:

> The structure of community involvement changed. We used to meet in the evening because the majority of the people were activists that had

our own jobs. When the Ryan White CARE Act came into being, a lot of the [activists] moved to work at larger organizations or at the public agencies, because more positions became available with more funding. All of a sudden, those meetings that used to take place at 6 or 6:30 were taking place at 9 in the morning. That's the reason I left my job. It was very difficult for me to ask for permission to leave my work [in order to attend these meetings during the day]. It came to the point where if I wanted to continue to lead, I would have to be present at those meetings. If you're not present, you're not taken into consideration.

These AIDS organizations were limping along with scant resources until the 1990s. When a lot of money suddenly appeared on what used to be a very small table, it attracted many more people who rightfully wanted a place at that table. Noel Alumit argued that some activism remained, but it was of a different quality. It had become what he called "a place at the table" activism, constantly asking, "What about us? Where's our funding?" If people like Oscar and Dean were not in the room, their organizations (and the communities they served) would not even get scraps.

Over time, Noel became acclimated to this way of thinking. As he became one of the longest-serving staff at APAIT, he acknowledged, "There were younger activists who were coming in [as staff] and they wanted to rebel, to blow up the world [metaphorically] because it was unfair. Then I would say, 'Well, actually, no. There's an order that we need to fill at this time.' I think they might have been disappointed by that."

The shift from activism to professionalism was therefore in response to the structural changes in the way we funded the movement. People such as Oscar and Dean, the "reluctant" leaders, were perfectly content being the volunteers in the movement. But when the movement became the industry, either they had to get paid to play or they became irrelevant. Even leaders in ACT UP/LA, an activist-oriented group that would never consider public money to do direct services, began to take up these new staff positions in the expanded government bureaucracies. In a way, AIDS funding rang the death knell for many volunteer activist groups.

Not every organization succeeded in this transition. Oscar recalled that several Latino AIDS organizations that were around in the late

1980s along with Bienestar professionalized, got more funding, but eventually faltered. He said, "It wasn't that they weren't providing good services to the community. If we go back and look at what happened, it was all around their administrative audits that they didn't pass, cash flow that they didn't have. We have lots of heart, but we also need to pass program and financial audits."

Shawn Griffin of the Gay Men of Color Consortium added, "White agencies dot the i's and cross the t's. Communities of color weren't used to dealing with that type of structure. They would say, the most important thing is, when somebody comes in the door, they feel welcome, not that we're filling out all of this paperwork in the back." The bureaucracy's reliance on legal and administrative expertise was arguably a vestige of White supremacy, especially when you consider which communities were historically kept from developing that expertise through discrimination in higher education, employment or promotion, or how many leaders of color, once they were trained to develop that expertise in these marginalized organizations, were poached by their mainstream counterparts, foundations, or government agencies. The "brain drain" was then used to justify why these smaller organizations in communities of color could not compete for funding.

With his experience in an accounting office, Oscar had learned the importance of fiscal controls and administrative procedures. Nowadays, Bienestar operates as a community clinic in seven locations. Along with this growth spurt, Oscar had gotten "a lot of criticism that [he] had lost touch with the community." He said, "They would equate professionalization with not being grassroots anymore. How do you balance the need for community passion with organizational responsibility to your funders? That was a conversation we also had at the Gay Men of Color Consortium meetings. I believe merging the two was one of our hardest growing pains."

Even Joël, who had not much patience for institutionalization, had his reckoning moment. He had left LA to work for another Asian American health organization in the Bay Area. His mentors became these radical women who had roots in the Asian American movement during the 1970s, like Sherry Hirota, then CEO of Asian Health Services in Oakland:

> They were like my mother's sisters, and they recognized me, and they said, "Oh, you're a trouble-maker." Sherry said, "I know your

reputation. That's why we're going to train you." They were like, "Yeah, yeah, yeah, we know your values. You're not the first one. Yeah, yeah, yeah, you're so radical. Yeah, yeah, yeah, you're so innovative. But do you know how to do a budget? This is how you do a budget, and this is how you do program planning, and this is what evaluation is, and this is how you deal with staff, and this is how you deal with public funds." It was straight-up boot camp and it still informs my life now. I remember their words: "It's not about you being an office lackey. It's about you being able to do movement work [inside the system]. You need technical skills. So shut the fuck up and learn it." To them, I listened. At that time no one could tell me to shut the fuck up, but Sherry Hirota could tell me to this day to shut the fuck up and I will have to listen.

As Joël reflected on those years, he realized, "I also became less radical as I got older and my salary got bigger. When I started to having to manage people, I thought, 'Okay, you don't get to be the enfant terrible anymore. You have to put in like the rest of us.' That's when I actually felt a pretty marked shift." This shift included going back to school. Joël had been "a big fuck-you to Academia up until [his] late twenties." Having cofounded organizations and published works that college students would read in their classes, Joël thought Academia was going to "ruin [his] voice." Then in his thirties, he said, "Some of my mentees would come back to the field and they would sign off on my projects because they had the credentials." The field had professionalized to the point that his years of experience could no longer substitute for having alphabets after his name, when people he'd trained were now overseeing his work. Professionalism was going to turn him into a "dinosaur"—unless he did something about it. "My immigrant mother was right," he concluded. "I should get my fucking degree. My immigrant kicked in. I was like 'You'd better get your degree. And you'd better get it from a good institution, dummy.'" He went on to graduate from UC Berkeley.

With professionalization, APAIT also began to attract Asian American celebrities in the entertainment industry to help pitch its fundraising. Amy Hill, the *hapa* actor who had developed a following even before her turn as Margaret Cho's grandmother in the pioneering but short-lived

TV show *All-American Girl* (1994–95), was one of the earliest APAIT sup-
porters. In 1995, Hill dedicated the opening night of her one-woman
show *Reunion* in Hollywood to be APAIT's first major fundraiser. The
show about Hill's mother, a Japanese war bride in South Dakota, netted
over $5,000 to the agency and attracted corporate sponsors, such as ABC
(which aired *All-American Girl*) and community partners, including
AIDS Healthcare Foundation and APLA.

Healthier Solutions, Robert Berger's firm, was also a sponsor. Robert leveraged his Hollywood connections to garner another fundraiser
for APAIT in the following year. His friend Elizabeth Sung, a rare
Asian American actress on the daytime soap opera *The Young and the
Restless*, was part of the Directing Workshop for Women at the American Film Institute. Under Sung's direction and with a script she cowrote
with her husband, the film *Requiem*, which starred Tamlyn Tomita and
Chris Hashima, told the story of Sung's brother Philip, a fashion
designer who died of AIDS in 1985. Robert produced the film's premiere
at the Academy of Television Arts and Sciences and arranged it to be a
fundraiser for APAIT. In a 1995 profile in the *Los Angeles Times,* Sung
described her brand of AIDS resistance as "a quiet activism." She said,
"I'm hoping my version of activism will help bring a certain awareness
to people who may be careless, so they'll take care of themselves better"
(figure 18.1). The premiere event was anything but quiet. Close to three
hundred people attended the event, a mixture of APAIT clients, Hollywood celebrities, and corporate sponsors (like Pacific Bell, Wells
Fargo, and Kaiser Permanente). Philip Moon, Sung's costar on *The Young
and the Restless*, and Amy Hill emceed the event. The screening also featured live performances by homegrown artists Leilani Chan, Ke'o
Woolford, and APAIT's own Napoleon Lustre.[1]

Few events showed the tension between the radical beginnings of
the Asian American AIDS movement and its mainstreaming more than
this event. Napoleon had often incorporated smoking a cigarette as part
of his act. He explained, "They were always non-smoking spaces and I
was pissed off. So I'd make it part of the act, and they would have to say
yes." Perhaps in defiance of the posh academy setting, Napoleon—on a
"spur of the moment"—ground the burning cigarette into his arm. During our interview, he showed me the scar from that performance, which
he had since enclosed in a biohazard tattoo, the symbol that many

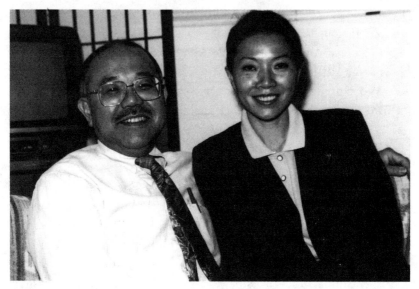

FIGURE 18.1. APAIT director Dean Goishi with actress Elizabeth Sung. Courtesy of Robert Berger.

HIV-positive people wore to signal pride and solidarity with one another. At the event, the denouement punctuated Napoleon's sobering performance about his unending confrontation with death, but the audience found it uncomfortable and distressing. In the debrief of the event, Robert reported that some even found it "offensive."

This controversy aside, the AIDS cause was becoming not just mainstream in the 1990s, but downright respectable. Even the LA Philharmonic got into the act in 1998. As J Craig Fong, the first chair of APAIT's advisory board, recalled:

> I had a friend who was a musician. She put me in touch with the Asian members of the philharmonic. Interestingly, at the time, they were all strings. I don't know what stereotype that says. We sat down and I said, "Even if it's just a string quartet, even if there are just four of you who are willing to step forward to this tiny little organization, we could rent a room and sell $50 a ticket." This isn't Madonna. This isn't Cher. This isn't some gay icon. It's the very respectable LA Phil, and they're doing a string concert, so our Asian American parents could come. And the Asian organizations, restaurants, supermarkets, who

might have been afraid to be attached to a fundraiser for gay people, would promote it. It gave them a respectability. I hate that word, but it gave them a cover that was not so openly gay and lesbian to support it.

The first year, eight musicians volunteered for the event. The number of performers would grow in subsequent years. In 2000, the concert was held at the historic Biltmore Hotel. Even the non-Asian musicians on the orchestra wanted to pitch in.

J acknowledged "a generational difference," in that events like this targeted a different milieu than the typical APAIT client. "You can have a fundraiser for old fogies like me," he said, "for the more established organizations, the stores and whatnot. That doesn't mean six months later you can't have something that's more for the younger club crowd, something less stuffy."

The AIDS movement, for better or for worse, had grown up.

The medicalization of the epidemic also contributed to the waning of the movement. Short of a cure, the advent of the protease inhibitors in the mid-1990s complemented earlier drugs—into what many people called the "cocktail"—and improved treatment outcomes for many people living with HIV. Tracy said, "Our clients were doing a lot better. People that went on disability before were now able to return to work." Hospices were closing. People who had felt like they were living with a timebomb now had to think about a future. Some had racked up debts that they thought they would not live long enough to have to repay. Having survived the epidemic, they had to deal with the grief and guilt over those who hadn't. As they got older, they began to worry about all the other chronic conditions that came with aging. As one of them said, "Good news is you're living longer. Bad news is you're living longer."

When Gil Mangaoang found out in his early forties that he was HIV positive, he and his partner, Juan Lombard, gave themselves "seven years to make the most of what we wanted to do." Then seven years passed. He was still alive and turning fifty. His health wasn't always good, but HIV wasn't the death sentence it once was. What did they do? They bought a condo and got married on the roof, overlooking the LA skylines. "We've been together now with him being HIV positive longer than not being," Juan added. "It's almost like dealing with somebody who has diabetes."

Even without a cure—and exactly because we don't have a cure—AIDS medications proved to be a boon to the pharmaceutical companies. They even found a way to profit from healthy people. In 2012, the FDA approved pre-exposure prophylaxis (PrEP) to keep HIV-negative people from getting the virus. Unlike a one-time vaccine, these antiviral drugs have to be taken daily. This is not to say that these advances were a setback. Many people have been able to live longer because of them, and untold many will not contract the virus. The fact remains, the struggle that captured so much imagination of a generation of queer activists decades before has become a biomedical saga, out of the hands of grassroots activists and people with HIV. There is just an iota of emphasis on overhauling the health-care system. They became part of that system. Many current AIDS service organizations could survive only after they transformed into community clinics. Bienestar is an example of this. In San Francisco, API Wellness Center, which was once an AIDS service organization serving the Asian community in the Bay Area, is now the San Francisco Community Health Center.

For a brief period during the 2010s, APAIT tried its hand at converting into a federally qualified health center but didn't quite find a foothold. It now capitalizes on a different strength. Recently, the agency deliberately aligns itself with emerging trans organizations in the city. These organizations, like Gender Justice LA and TransLatin@ Coalition, are co-located with the APAIT office in Koreatown. Some of their trans and gender non-conforming members became members of the APAIT staff. The Trans Wellness Center, a collaboration of six agencies—APAIT, Bienestar, Children's Hospital Los Angeles, Friends Community Center, the Los Angeles LGBT Center, and TransLatin@ Coalition—is located on the same floor as APAIT. It offers housing, employment, benefits enrollment, legal, mental health, and sexual health services for people who identify as trans or gender non-binary. In 2019, APAIT, in a collaboration with another Special Service for Groups division focusing on homelessness, acquired a house in Koreatown that would provide bridge housing to homeless trans women, a first of its kind in LA County. The sixteen-bed house, Casa de Zulma, is named after the late trans activist and former APAIT staff member Zulma Velasquez, who died just months before the house was open. Bigger than ever—and now with an office in the adjacent Orange County—APAIT still managed to cling to its principles of innovation, collaboration, and advocacy for those most invisible in our society, even when operating in a highly regulative environment.

But as Tracy Nako observed at the end of our interview, there is now no mention of "Asian" or "Pacific Islander" in APAIT's mission. The agency was still led by an Asian American director, Jury Candelario, but the majority of its staff, while predominantly people of color, was no longer Asian. The trajectory of the epidemic, including the funding to fight it, has over the years taken the agency to a different frontier. Yet the current agency has its roots in the movement from those early years—multiracial coalition was a hallmark of APAIT's advocacy—even if it is not recognizable to those who kept it plodding along in that formative time.

Epilogue

A MOVEMENT IS NEVER FUTILE SIMPLY BECAUSE IT FADES INTO THE mainstream. The raw energies that ignited a movement may be curbed by its newly institutionalized incarnation, and its once-fringe messages may now be toned down as others become their torchbearers. Yet when a movement, in its push against the mainstream, moves the center of our political discourse toward liberation, this in itself is a marked success

Lisa Hasegawa told me, "I've always felt like the folks in the HIV/AIDS community in the API [Asian Pacific Islander] world have been leading Asian American advocacy for the past twenty years. You can connect a lot of the leadership back to those early days of advocacy around HIV/AIDS." She cited people such as Ignatius Bau, Gem Daus, Suki Terada Ports—and stopped before she realized she'd inevitably leave out someone in the long list she was compiling in her head. Even Lisa herself, recognized as a national leader with her time as the executive director at National Coalition for Asian Pacific American Community Development, said, "I certainly connect my introduction to advocacy to HIV/AIDS organizing." This far-reaching impact of the Asian American AIDS movement on broader advocacy for the Asian American community was seldom acknowledged.

For my generation, these activists reclaimed sex that was rendered deadly by the virus and demonized by conservatives. In so doing, they validated an essential part of our human experience. The AIDS movement showed that sex is a legitimate principle on which to build a social movement—a pleasure principle, if you will. Few other progressive movements were built on this human condition.

When I taught a course in Asian American studies on gender and sexuality, I began the term by assigning Linda España Maram's book, *Creating Masculinity in Los Angeles's Little Manila: Working-Class Filipinos and Popular Culture, 1920s–1950s*. For a course that was ostensibly about non-normative gender and sexual identities, some students and colleagues (even Maram herself) were befuddled by this choice. The *manongs* in Maram's book were as conventionally heterosexual as they came. There are many books about that generation of Filipino migrant workers in the US, and almost all of them predictably focus on their subject's identity as laborers. After all, Asian American studies has historically been a political project to reclaim the lives of early immigrants who came to this country to fill a labor niche after the abolition of slavery. In this historical reclamation, these scholars justify the contributions of these early immigrants and challenge the assumption that our republic was founded on Whiteness, a manifest destiny. But this reclamation is *our* political project. What I appreciated about Maram's work was that she centered the lives of these early immigrants in how they would define themselves. The hard manual labor that built this country was what they had to do to survive. It wasn't the essence of who they were. That essence was in their gender and sexual expression; they would rather be defined by those things that Maram talked about in her book: dancing (mostly with White women) in taxi dance halls, donning elaborate zoot suits that they spent much of their hard-earned money on, and going to boxing matches for a chance to see a Brown body emerge victorious. Like our academic disciplines, our social movements generally do not concern themselves with the idea of pleasure, even though it is a major principle that governs our relationships, our life decisions, and our joy. Especially in the 1970s, LGBTQ activists in leftist communities of color had to separate—no, excise—that part of themselves in order to be taken seriously by their movement comrades. AIDS activism changed all that. These activists did not ask for permission bashfully. They stood firm in their position that no matter how you decide to live your life and find joy, you deserve a home and a community. And even in the throes of despair from a relentless epidemic, we will not give up that joy.

Nowadays, young people who do not subscribe to the gender binary embrace their non-conforming appearance in public. They force mainstream institutions, like hotels and universities, to turn their facilities gender neutral. They are living a queerness that many in our generation were only dreaming of and theorizing. I am drawing a through line between the uber-straight *manongs* at the turn of the twentieth century and these brave young activists, with the AIDS movement right smack in the middle.

For me and the AIDS activists I talked to, now in our middle age, it is easy to succumb to the romance of our youth as "those golden days." Yet I didn't take on this project to reclaim a comforting sense of nostalgia. Those days were far from perfect. That these activists were flawed human beings doing the best they could endears them to me more than if they were master strategists who knew every next step along the way. Their collective stories impart something essential about movement building that is still relevant today. Ultimately, this movement is a story of youth, who charted their course in a way that made sense to them, even when sometimes it meant pissing off an older generation that had more experience. J Craig Fong analogized this youthful energy as yeast to bread: "If you want a loaf of bread to rise, you need some yeast. Every organization needs a few perhaps less-than-easy-to-handle people, people who are a little too outspoken, who are a little too impatient, who maybe lack the memory of the people who came before." The young, mostly queer, Asian American activists in the early AIDS movement might not have had much of a blueprint, but they did draw their ideas from a deep well of radical feminists of color and from explicit and uncompromising writers and artists. From them, they might not have learned specific tactics, but they learned something far more useful and sustaining: boldness, inventiveness, irreverence, intersectionality, and a sense of justice for the most marginalized. These, I believe, are the building blocks of any movement.

As I guide these stories to young activists today, I wish to tell them, take whatever you find useful from this lineage, and ditch the rest. Make your mistakes and learn from them, no apologies necessary. Don't let people from my generation tell you otherwise. Even if we had known better, that was a different time and place.

This is your world now.

NOTES

CHAPTER 1: BRAND NEW WORLD

1 Mangaoang, "From the 1970s to the 1990s," 40.
2 Julie V. Iovine, "'Lipsticks' and Lords: Yale's New Look," *Wall Street Journal*, August 4, 1987; Nick Ravo, "Yale President Rebuts Story that Depicted School as 'Gay.'" *New York Times*, September 29, 1987.

CHAPTER 2: UNIVERSAL PRECAUTIONS

1 "Another Bigot Named Pat," *Bay Area Reporter* 26, no. 8 (February 22, 1996); "Dems to Pick New National, State Bosses," *Bay Area Reporter* 19, no. 3 (January 19, 1989).
2 "AIDS: No to Hysteria," *Los Angeles Times*, August 13, 1985; Mark Star with David L. Gonzalez, "The Panic over AIDS," *Newsweek*, July 4, 1983.
3 "Morticians Refused to Embalm 80-Year-Old AIDS Victim," *Associated Press*, February 27, 1985.
4 "None of These Will Give You AIDS." Poster, Illinois Department of Public Health, 1987.
5 Frederick M. Muir, "Council Rejects AIDS Tests for Restaurant Workers," *Los Angeles Times*, December 12, 1991.
6 Stephen Braun, "Judge Rules against AIDS Patient in Suit over Pedicure Refusal," *Los Angeles Times*, April 24, 1987.
7 "Few Dentists for Patients with AIDS." *USA Today*, July 20, 1987.
8 Harry Nelson, "Doctors See No AIDS Link to Mannequins in CPR Classes," *Los Angeles Times*, June 18, 1983.

CHAPTER 3: A RUMOR OF PLAGUE

1 Choi et al., "Age and Race Mixing Patterns," 53.

CHAPTER 4: FUCK THAT

1 Roth, *The Life and Death of ACT UP/LA*, 106.

CHAPTER 6: SCHOOL OF FISH

1 Los Angeles County AIDS Commission, Meeting Minutes, August 13, 1987. ONE National Gay & Lesbian Archives, University of Southern California, Los Angeles, California.

2 Los Angeles County AIDS Commission, Meeting Minutes, November 20, 1987. ONE National Gay & Lesbian Archives, University of Southern California, Los Angeles, California.

3 Named after the African American physician who pioneered blood preservation until he was tragically killed in an auto accident in 1950, the Charles R. Drew Medical Society has a mission to "promote the interests of physicians and patients of African descent" and to be a "leading voice" for "the elimination of health disparities."

4 Doug Sadownick, "The AIDS Community in LA," *LA Weekly*, November 25–December 1, 1988.

5 Asian Pacific AIDS Intervention Team, Board Retreat, September 16, 1995. APAIT archives.

6 Sadownick, "The AIDS Community in LA."

CHAPTER 8: FILTHY, DIRTY ADS

1 Nguyen, *A View from the Bottom*, 155.

2 Nguyen, *A View from the Bottom*, 244n8.

CHAPTER 11: WE WANT A NEW DRUG

1 Alice Park, "The Story behind the First AIDS Drug," *Time*, March 19, 2017.

2 Bruce Lambert, "AIDS Insurance Coverage Is Increasingly Hard to Get," *New York Times,* August 7, 1989.

3 Milt Freudenheim, "AZT Maker Expected to Reap Big Gain," *New York Times*, August 19, 1989; Victor F. Zonana, "AIDS Groups Urge Firm to Lower AZT Price," *Los Angeles Times*, August 31, 1989; Marilyn Chase, "Wellcome

PLC Sets Price of AIDS Drug at $8,300 a Year, Higher than Expected," *Wall Street Journal*, February 7, 1987.

4 Michael Spector, "Pressure from AIDS Activists Has Transformed Drug Testing," *Washington Post*, July 2, 1989.

5 Margie Patlak, "The Arsenal Gets Larger," *Discover,* April 1989.

6 Joshua Hammer, "The AIDS Underground: Herbs, Hormones and Smuggling Runs Overseas," *Newsweek*, August 7, 1989

7 Alex Keown, "Companies Fight for Growing Share of HIV Market," Biospace, May 1, 2018, www.biospace.com/article/companies-fight-for-growing-share-of-hiv-market.

CHAPTER 12: THAT SHRINKING WINDOW OF RECONCILIATION

1 Kameya and Kameya, "A Parent's Perspective."

CHAPTER 17: NOT TO BE DICKED AROUND

1 Schwartz, "New Alliances, Strange Bedfellows," 230–31.

2 Schwartz, "New Alliances, Strange Bedfellows," 231.

3 Roth, *The Life and Death of ACT UP/LA*, 94.

CHAPTER 18: DOWNRIGHT RESPECTABLE

1 N. F. Mendoza, "With an Eye on . . . : Loss of Her Brother Puts Soap Star Elizabeth Sung on a Quietly Active Path," *Los Angeles Times*, May 28, 1995.

BIBLIOGRAPHY

Choi, Kyung-Hee, et al. "Age and Race Mixing Patterns of Sexual Partnerships among Asian Men Who Have Sex with Men: Implications for HIV Transmission and Prevention." *AIDS Education and Prevention* 15, no. 1 (Supplement, 2003): 53–65.

Clough, Juliana, Sunmin Lee, and David H. Chae. "Barriers to Health Care among Asian Immigrants in the United States: A Traditional Review." *Journal of Health Care for the Poor and Underserved* 24, no. 1 (2013): 384–403.

España-Maram, Linda. *Creating Masculinity in Los Angeles's Little Manila: Working-Class Filipinos and Popular Culture, 1920s–1950s.* New York: Columbia University Press, 2006.

Farber, Celia. "Sins of Omission: The AZT Scandal." *Spin*, November 1989.

Gadsby, Patricia. "The Virus Strikes Back." *Discover*, July 1989.

Han, C. Winter. *Geisha of a Different Kind: Race and Sexuality in Gaysian America.* New York: New York University Press, 2015.

Ho, Man Keung. "Applying Family Therapy Theories to Asian/Pacific Americans." *Contemporary Family Therapy* 11, no. 1 (1989): 61–70.

Hom, Alice Y. "Stories from the Homefront: Perspectives of Asian American Parents with Lesbian Daughters and Gay Sons." *Amerasia Journal* 20, no. 1 (1994): 19–32.

Hsiao, An-Fu, Mitchell D. Wong, Michael S. Goldstein, Lida S. Becerra, Eric M. Cheng, and Neil S. Wenger. "Complementary and Alternative Medicine Use among Asian-American Subgroups: Prevalence, Predictors, and Lack of Relationship to Acculturation and Access to Conventional Health Care." *Journal of Alternative and Complementary Medicine* 12, no. 10 (2006): 1003–10.

Jung, E. Alex. "The Big Queer Universe of Gregg Araki: The Filmmaker on *Now Apocalypse,* Writing through the AIDS Crisis and Trump Era, and Gay-Baiting on *Riverdale." Vulture,* March 21, 2019.

Kameya, Harold, and Ellen Kameya. "A Parent's Perspective: Give Back Our Daughter's Right to Marry." Asian & Friends Denver, June 4, 2010. www .afdenver.net/forparents.php.

Kenney, Moira. *Mapping Gay LA: The Intersection of Place and Politics.* Philadelphia: Temple University Press, 2001.

Lee, Deborah A., and Kevin Fong. "HIV/AIDS and the Asian and Pacific Islander Community." *SIECUS Report* 18, no. 3 (1990): 16–22.

Lee, Sunmin, Genevieve Martinez, Grace X. Ma, Chiehwen E. Hsu, E. Stephanie Robinson, Julie Bawa, and Hee-Soon Juon. "Barriers to Health Care Access in 13 Asian American Communities." *American Journal of Health Behavior* 34, no. 1 (2010): 21–30.

Mangaoang, Gil. "From the 1970s to the 1990s: Perspective of a Gay Filipino American Activist." *Amerasia Journal* 20, no. 1 (1994): 33–44.

Masequesmay, Gina. "Everyday Identity Works at an Asian Pacific AIDS Organization." In *Cultural Compass: Ethnographic Explorations of Asian America*, edited by Martin Manalansan IV, 113–38. Philadelphia: Temple University Press, 2000.

Nguyen, Tan Hoang. *A View from the Bottom: Asian American Masculinity and Sexual Representation.* Durham, NC: Duke University Press, 2014.

Omatsu, Glenn. "The 'Four Prisons' and the Movements of Liberation: Asian American Activism from the 1960s and the 1990s." In *The State of Asian America: Activism and Resistance in the 1990s,* edited by Karin Aguilar-San Juan, 19–69. Boston: South End Press, 1994.

Ordoña, Trinity A. "Asian Lesbians in San Francisco: Struggles to Create a Safe Space, 1970s–1980s." In *Asian/Pacific Islander American Women: A Historical Anthology*, edited by Shirley Hune and Gail M. Nomura, 319–34. New York: New York University Press, 2003.

Parish, Ric, James Sakakura, Brian Green, Joël B. Tan, and Robert Vàzquez Pacheco. "Communion: A Collaboration on AIDS." In *Asian American Sexualities: Dimensions of the Gay & Lesbian Experience*, edited by Russell Leong, 201–17. New York: Routledge, 1996.

Richman, Douglas D., Margaret A. Fischl, Michael H. Grieco, Michael S. Gottlieb, Paul A. Volberding, Oscar L. Laskin, John M. Leedom, et al. "The Toxicity of Azidothymidine (AZT) in the Treatment of Patients with AIDS and AIDS-Related Complex." *New England Journal of Medicine* 317, no. 4 (1987): 192–97.

Roth, Benita. *The Life and Death of ACT UP/LA: Anti-AIDS Activism in Los Angeles from the 1980s to the 2000s.* New York: Cambridge University Press, 2017.

Schulman, Sarah. *Gentrification of the Mind: Witness to a Lost Imagination.* Berkeley: University of California Press, 2012.

Schwartz, Ruth. "New Alliances, Strange Bedfellows: Lesbians, Gay Men, and AIDS." In *Sisters, Sexperts, Queers: Beyond the Lesbian Nation*, edited by Arlene Stein, 230–44. New York: Plume, 1993.

Tung, Wei-Chen. "Asian American's Confucianism-Based Health-Seeking Behavior and Decision-Making Process." *Home Health Care Management & Practice* 22, no. 7 (2010): 536–38.

Wat, Eric C. "Preserving the Paradox: Stories from a Gay-Ioh." *Amerasia Journal* 20, no. 1 (1994): 149–60.

———. *The Making of a Gay Asian Community: An Oral History of Pre-AIDS Los Angeles.* New York: Rowman & Littlefield, 2002.

INDEX

AIDS Project Los Angeles (APLA)
(*continued*)
Sally Jue as first Asian American staff
at, 29; Tracy Nako and, 104
AIDS quilt, 221
AIDS service demonstration grants
(HRSA), 88, 89
Alfaro, Luis, 119
All-American Girl (ABC), 257
Altamed, 90
Alumit, Noel, 98*fig.*; Abbey magnet
event, 114; Boy Toy controversy
and, 237, 239, 242; on club outreach,
106; on coming out and AIDS,
25–26; county outreach contract
and, 129; on dating, 195–97; on gay
artists and mentors, 110; on grief,
210–11; Highways and, 119; on
James Sakakura, 220; on "place at
the table" activism, 254; profile,
96–99; "A Question of Parity"
conference and, 233–34; social
marketing campaigns and, 132–34,
139; on women with AIDS, 231
American Psychiatric Association
(APA), 21, 37–38
API Parents and Friends of Lesbians
and Gays, 184
API Wellness Center, San Francisco,
260
Araki, Gregg, 120
Arnau, Darryl, 130–31, 134
"Asian American," as term, 10, 21
Asian American Advertising and
Public Relations Alliance, 137
Asian American Drug Abuse Program
(AADAP), 29–30, 41, 104, 173
"Asian and Pacific Islander" (API), as
term, 9–10
Asian culture. *See* cultural issues, Asian

Asian Pacific AIDS Education Project:
Dean Goishi and, 42–44, 56–61; Eric
Reyes and, 59, 69, 247; formation of,
42–44; funding and leadership of,
56–61, 69; GMOCC and, 91;
translation services grant, 82
Asian Pacific AIDS Intervention Team
(APAIT): in twenty-first century,
260–61; artists and writers on staff,
113–14; bathhouse outreach, 103;
Boy Toy controversy and, 235–38;
buddy program, 144–46; Casa de
Zulma, 260; case management,
104–5, 146–49, 151; club outreach,
105–6; counseling services, 173–76,
179–82; dayroom, 149–51, 221; Diep
Tran and, 192–94; divisions,
249–50; ethnic-specific organizations and cosponsored social
events, 185–86; founding of, 4, 11,
68–69; fraternization policy,
196–99; generational shift, 93–94;
GMOCC and, 83, 86–88, 91–92;
hiring criteria and political/creative
early staff, 244–46; illness and
mental health among staff, 210–11;
James Sakakura and, 217–22; J
Craig Fong and, 78–79; Keith Kasai
and, 171–72; LAAPIS and, 190–91;
LA Philharmonic fundraiser,
258–59; Margaret Endo Shimada at,
30; Napoleon Lustre profile,
99–103; Noel Alumit profile,
96–99; prevention case management, 198; prevention outreach and
messaging, 107–9; *Requiem* film
premiere fundraiser, 257–58;
sensitivity training, 192–93; sex
education program, 124; South
Asian Outreach Task Force,

CARE (Ryan White Comprehensive AIDS Resources Emergency) Act (1990), 88–91, 194, 224, 253–54

caregiving by activists, 202–5

Casa de Zulma, 260

case management: APAIT and, 104–5, 146–49, 151; prevention case management, 198

Castro, Marissa, 59

Centers for Disease Control and Prevention (CDC), 24

Chan, Leilani, 257

Charles R. Drew Medical Society, 71, 266n3(ch6)

Chikahisa, Paul, 61, 65

Chin, Douglas, 36, 65

Chin, Justin, 119

Chinese medicine, traditional, 157, 160

Chinese Rainbow Association, 184

Chingusai, 184, 186

Cho, Margaret, 256–57

Choi, Kyung-Hee, 34

Choksey, Rashmi, 189

Chow, Prescott, 129

Chris Brownlie Hospice, 97–98

Christenson, Kim, 127

Christianity and homophobia, 5

Chun, Eileen, 136

Clinton, Bill, 94

Colors United Action Coalition, 53–54, 64

coming out: 1970s liberalization and, 21; in age of AIDS, 96; community groups and, 185–86; cultural barriers, layers of, 179–80; Dean Goishi and, 44–45; Diep Tran and, 191–92; Dredge Kang and, 128; family reactions to AIDS vs., 169–70; forced by AIDS, 182; Gil Mangaoang and, 13–14, 15;

homophobia, parents, and, 177; James Sakakura and, 213–14; Keith Kasai and, 168–70, 177; LGBTQ-specific spaces and, 183; Noel Alumit on AIDS and, 25–26; normalization and, 142; P-FLAG and, 178, 184; Ric Parish and, 23; Valerie Kameya and, 177

Compound Q , 155

condoms, 107, 108–9

Corpus, Peter, 236–37, 242

counseling: APAIT counseling services, 173–76, 179–82; bereavement, 29; grief counseling, 211; for HIV test results, 19–20

couples' therapy, 175

Course in Miracles, A (Schucman), 155

Creating Masculinity in Los Angeles's Little Manila (Maram), 263

Crisostomo, Vince, 129

Cuffs Bar, 202–3

cultural capital, 246

cultural competence, 5, 37, 228

cultural issues, Asian: coming out, layers of barriers to, 179–80; death and dying, embarrassment over, 37, 187; denial of homosexuality and HIV/AIDS, 26, 33–34, 40, 43, 139; homophobia and, 4–5; messages in red envelopes and fortune cookies, 108–9; underreporting and, 80–81

cytomegalovirus retinitis, 159

D

dating, 195–201

Daus, Gem, 262

dayroom (APAIT), 149–51

de la O, Oscar: on APLA, 73; GMOCC and, 84, 86–87, 91–92; on ill GLLU

Gay Asian Pacific Support Network (GAPSN) (*continued*) formation of, 184; Noel Alumit and, 196–97; social events, 191

Gay Asian Rap Group (GARP), 183–84

Gay Men of Color Consortium (GMOCC), 83–92, 255

Gay Vietnamese Alliance, 184

gender and sexism: AIDS funding for women, lack of, 224–25; APAIT hiring of women, 227–30; Boy Toy controversy, 234–43; deference, sexism disguised as, 228–29; gay men and sexism, 223; health care, bias in, 161–62, 231. *See also* women

Gender Justice LA, 260

Gerald, Gilberto, 87

Gilead, 165

Glaxo Wellcome, 165

Gock, Terry: AIT and, 38–42, 60, 67; background, 37–38; as clinician, 174; LA County AIDS Commission and, 74, 79; on selling prevention, 82

Goishi, Dean, 32*fig.*, 258*fig.*; APHCV and, 61–62; A/PLG and, 31–39, 60; APPCON and, 39–44; Asian Pacific AIDS Education Project and, 42–44, 56–61; Boy Toy controversy and, 237; California Community Foundation grant and, 42; caregiving and, 202–3; client testimonial letter sent to, 150; as face of HIV in Asian American community, 44–45; fraternization and, 197; GMOCC and, 85, 86–87, 92; grief and, 208–11; growth management and, 246–49; on hiring criteria, 244; HIV Planning Council and, 90; interview with, 10; James Sakakura and,

218, 221; J Craig Fong and, 78–79; Kameyas and, 177; on "Love Your Asian Body" campaign, 121; public speaking and, 83; "A Question of Parity" conference and, 233; Sally Jue and, 30; social marketing campaigns and, 139; softer side of, 211; staff and, 104, 128, 129, 137, 173–74, 199; Tom Callahan and, 202–5, 208–9; women staff and, 224, 227–30

Goldberg, Whoopi, 101

Great Leap, 111–12, 112*fig.*

Green, Brian, 214, 215

grief, 15, 205–11, 220–22

Griffin, Shawn: on APAIT, 87; on bureaucracy, 255; *Edge* article, 85–86; "Love Your Asian Body" campaign and, 123; on reaction to HIV, 26; treatment advocacy and, 158, 161

growth management, 246–49

H

Harbor/UCLA Medical Center, 28

Harold, Larry, 91

Hasegawa, Lisa, 57–58, 61–64, 95, 109, 262

Hatanaka, Herb, 43, 65–66, 137, 138

health care: AIDS panic and the medical profession, 26–30; ambulance companies, discrimination by, 28–29; prevention vs. treatment, 92; race and access to, 54–55; sensitivity training, 192–93; sexism in, 161–62, 231; universal, 55; women's issues vs. AIDS funding, 224–25. *See also* treatment advocacy; treatments

Healthier Solutions, 136, 257–58

health insurance and drug costs, 153

Health Resources and Service
Administration (HRSA), 88
Helms Amendment, 75–76
herbal medicine, 157
Highways Performance Space, 119
Hill, Amy, 111–12, 256–57
Hirota, Sherry, 255–56
HIV: ban on immigrants with, 75–76;
dating and prejudice against,
199–201; incidence rates, 71, 79–82;
sexual orientation vs. HIV status,
169–70; stigma and, 4; women,
incidence rates among, 139; women,
risks to, 226–27. *See also* AIDS;
testing for HIV
HIV Health Services Planning
Councils, 89–90
Ho, David, 234
Hoffman, William, 96
Holden, Nate, 25
holistic medicine, 157, 160
Hom, Alice Y.: APAIT and, 228–29;
Boy Toy controversy and, 237, 240;
Highways and, 119; on lesbians and
HIV, 227; sexual exploration by, 22
homophobia: AIDS education and,
57–58; AIDS phobia and, 38; Asian
cultures and, 4–5, 57; Christianity
and, 5, 57–58; ethnic presses and,
134; families and, 170, 177–82;
internalized, 230; sensitivity
training and, 192; sex education
and, 123; strategies for fighting, 183;
substance abuse and, 41; virus,
comparison to, 177
homosexuality: as "abnormal" or
mental illness, 21, 24, 38; denial of,
in ethnic communities, 26, 33–34,
43, 187. *See also* coming out
Hudson, Rock, 88

I

Ibañez, Florante, 59
identity, lesbian and gay, 21–22
immigrants: APAIT, attraction of, 151;
APHCV and, 56; approach toward
immigrant communities, 4; Asian
American studies and, 263; Boy Toy
controversy and, 235–36, 242; case
management and, 147; concrete
assistance, need for, 150; difficulty
reaching, 3, 58–59, 77–78; educational outreach to, 58–59; ethnic
enclaves and, 6, 58, 234; ethnic-
specific organizations and, 184–90;
HIV ban, 75–76; mainstream vs.
ethnic providers and, 58; outreach
to reduce AIDS stigma, 135–36;
partnering within ethnic communities, 34–35; sexuality discussions
among, 141–42; SIPA and, 55; social
marketing and, 122, 131, 138; stories
of, 27–28, 38–39, 148–49, 206;
traditional medicine and, 80;
treatment advocacy and, 160–61;
underreporting and, 80–81. *See also*
Pacific Asian Language Services
(PALS)
immigration policy, 74–79
immunity rumor, 33–35
India, 188
interleukin-2, 155

J

Jackson, Michael, 88–89
Japan, annual AIDS Day in, 218
Japanese American Citizens' League
(JACL), 184
Jivani, Mushtaque, 187
Joo, JJ, 63–64, 197–99, 200*fig.*, 241

Joo, Karen Kimura: background, 127–28; on gender, 224; James Sakakura and, 220; JJ Joo and, 197–99, 200*fig.*; restructuring and, 249–50; social marketing campaigns and, 131, 134–35, 138, 140

Jordan, Wilbert, 162–63

Joslin, Leo Y., 240

Jue, Sally: AADAP and, 173; AIT split from A/PLG and, 67; AIT workshops, 37; APLA and, 29, 72; A/PLG and, 30, 33, 59–60; APPCON and, 39–43; Boy Toy controversy and, 234–35, 237–42; as clinician, 174; on cultural stigma, 80; early AIDS case and, 27–29; on generational difference, 94; on grief, 207, 211; immigrants and, 58–59; on prevention funds, 82; sexism and, 223; as social worker, 225; on women as less threatening, 223–24

June 28th Union (San Francisco), 14

JUST, 184

K

Kageyama, Naomi: AIT split from A/PLG and, 65; "Facing HIV and AIDS" campaign and, 138, 140; funding proposals and, 60–61; on gender, 224; James Sakakura and, 221; Margaret Endo Shimada and, 173–74; recollections of, 82

Kalayaan Collective, 12

Kameya, Ellen, 177–79

Kameya, Harold, 177–79

Kameya, Valerie, 177–79

Kamiyama, Pauline, 149, 209–11, 227

Kang, Dredge, 217*fig.*; APAIT restructuring and, 249–53; background,

128–29; Boy Toy controversy and, 235, 241; community groups and, 185–86; James Sakakura and, 217; JJ Joo and, 198; *KoreAm Journal* and, 141–42; outreach approaches, 130; sex education and, 125; social marketing campaigns and, 129–32, 134–35; Tracy Nako and, 195; on women's programming, 231

Kang, Unhei: about, 94–96; Boy Toy controversy and, 236, 242; death threat and, 139; gender dynamics and, 225, 227, 230–31; on hiring criteria, 244; Karen Kimura and, 128; *KoreAm Journal* and, 141–42; LAAPIS and, 96, 190–91; "Love Your Asian Body" campaign and, 116, 117*fig.*, 118, 121; on outreach by women, 106; sex education and, 123–24

Kaposi's sarcoma, 158–59

Kaposi's Sarcoma Foundation, 72

Kasai, Keith, 114, 116, 155–56, 167–73, 176–79

Katipunan ng mga Demokratikong Pilipino (KDP), 12–18

Katz, Mark, 90

Kawasaki, Roy, 36

Kawata, Paul, 237

Keiro, 173

Kheir (Korean Health Education, Information, and Referrals), 42, 186

Kim, Jeff, 241

Kimura, Karen. *See* Joo, Karen Kimura

KoreAm Journal, 141–42

Korean Community Service Center, 129

Koryo Health Foundation, 57, 197–98

Kraus, Jerry Michael, 14–16

Kuramoto, Ford, 40–41

Kwong, Dan, 111–12

men who have sex with men (MSM) population (*continued*) organizations and, 185; funding for outreach to, 61, 129; incidence rates and, 34; professionalization and, 250; South Asian, 188–89; women activists and, 128; WSW, 227

Milburn, Brent, 18

Miller, Tim, 119

Minority AIDS Project (MAP): Gilberto Gerald and, 87; GMOCC and, 83, 91; HIV Planning Council and, 90; LA County AIDS Commission and, 71, 74

Miyamoto, Nobuko, 111–13, 112*fig.*

model minority myth, 34, 252

monogamy, 17

Moon, Philip, 257

Morales, Royal (Uncle Roy), 40–41, 59

Morrison Hotel, 148

N

Nako, Tracy: about, 103–5; on APAIT as multiracial, 261; on camaraderie, 195; case management and, 104–5, 147–49; client-centered work and, 128; Commission on AIDS testimony, 80–81; on dating, 200; dayroom and, 149–51; on funding problems, 231; ill coworkers and, 210; JJ Joo and, 198; Keith Kasai and, 171; Margaret Endo Shimada and, 175; restructuring and, 249–50; tip on transgender hangout, 130

Narita, Jude, 111–12

National Coalition for Asian Pacific American Community Development, 262

National Gay and Lesbian Task Force, 54

National Minority AIDS Council, 233–34, 237

New Age approaches, 155

Nguyen, Long, 112–13

Nguyen Tan Hoang, 125–26

O

Office of AIDS, Los Angeles County, 42–43, 82, 92, 114–15, 150–51

Ogle, Albert, 74

Olivas, Arturo, 86

Omatsu, Glenn, 21

Ô-Môi, 184, 193–94, 229

Osato, Teri, 225

P

Pacific Asian Language Services (PALS) (SSG), 82, 135, 147–48, 233

parents. *See* family reactions

Parish, Ric, 50*fig.*; AB101 veto and, 48–49; on AIDS emergence, 23; AIT split from A/PLG and, 65–67; APAIT restructuring and, 250–52; A/PLG and, 61; Boy Toy controversy and, 235–39, 242; on club outreach, 106; dating protocol, 199–200; dayroom and, 149; on funding, 92; Karen Kimura and, 128; on Korean doctor, 26; "Love Your Asian Body" campaign and, 114–18, 121–23; Margaret Endo Shimada and, 175; on pharmaceutical companies, 165–66; taking over Joël Tan's job, 252; testing positive, 46–47; treatment advocacy and, 157–58, 160, 162–66; treatments and, 152, 156–57; Unhei Kang and, 95; on women with AIDS, 231

Park, Stephano, 186, 200–201
performance arts, 110–14, 124
Pets Are Wonderful Support (PAWS), 91
Pettit, Sarah, 22–23
P-FLAG (Parents and Friends of Lesbians and Gays), 177–78
pharmaceutical companies, 164–66, 260
pleasure, activist centering of, 5
PLUS (Positive Living for Us) seminar, 158
pneumocystis pneumonia (PCP), 28, 158–59
Ports, Suki Terada, 262
positive thinking, 155
Preston, Ashlee Marie, 55
Prevent AIDS Now Initiative Committee (PANIC), 25
prevention case management, 198
prevention efforts: APAIT prevention division, 249–50; Asian Pacific Islander outreach lagging, 11, 37; creative community building strategies, 245; focus on treatment vs., 91–92; funding for, 80, 81–82; Joël Tan, community spaces, and, 113; as outcome vs. activity, 185; outreach and messaging (APAIT), 107–9; self-esteem and, 121, 131–32; sexual explicitness and, 123–25; shift to high-risk populations, 60; women's programming (APAIT), 231–32. *See also* Asian Pacific AIDS Education Project; social marketing campaigns; testing for HIV
Pride parade, 171, 185, 194*fig.*
professionalization of APAIT: AIDS industry in general and, 253–55; early political and creative orientation, 244–46; Eric Reyes and, 247–48; fundraisers and, 256–59;

growth management and need for structure, 246–47; Joël Tan and, 255–56; restructuring into divisions, 249–53; staff growth and, 248–49
Project ABLE (AIDS Beliefs Learned through Education) (LA Free Clinic), 98
Project Ahead, 94
Proposition 64 (1986, CA), 25, 49, 84
protease inhibitors, 159, 259

Q

quarantine initiatives, 25, 49, 70, 84
Queer Nation, 48, 53–54, 120
"Question of Parity" conference (National Minority AIDS Council), 233–41

R

racism: APAIT restructuring and yellow colorism, 250–52; Boy Toy performance and blackface, 234–36, 242; cross-race sexual partnerships and, 35; health care access and, 54–55; internalized, 230; model minority myth, 34, 252. *See also* Whiteness and White Supremacy
Rafu Shimpo, 141, 172
Ransom, Alvin, 71
Reagan, Ronald, 45, 75–76, 196
Rebultan, Stanley, 156
red envelopes, 108–9
reproductive health education, 62–63
Requiem film premiere fundraiser, 257–58
Reunion (Hill), 257
Reyes, Eric: APAIT and, 93; Asian Pacific AIDS Education Project

Reyes, Eric (*continued*)
  and, 59, 69, 247; on Asian-White
  dynamic, 106–7; Colors United
  Action Coalition and, 53; Commission on AIDS testimony, 11; James
  Sakakura and, 221; "Love Your
  Asian Body" campaign and, 116, 118,
  121, 171; professionalization and,
  247–48; on sexism, 230–31; on
  women staff, 228
"rice queens," 33, 35, 120, 203
Riggs, Marlon, 119–20, 125
Rodriguez, Suzi, 90
Rosas, Crispin, 86
Roth, Benita, 48–49, 229, 232
Ryan White CARE Act (1990), 88–91,
  194, 224, 253–54

S

Sadownick, Doug, 72, 84
safer-sex outreach and presentations:
  at "Asian Night," 105; assembling
  kits as healing ritual, 211; cooking
  spoof, 126; LAAPIS, 191; messages
  in red envelopes and fortune
  cookies, 108–9; Phill Wilson and,
  123; by Sally Jue, 30; sexual
  explicitness in, 123–26
Safer Sex Sluts, 123–24
Sakakura, James, 217*fig.*; addiction and
  recovery, 215–16; at APAIT, 217;
  background and family life, 212–16;
  college and dropping out, 214–15;
  dayroom and, 149; dayroom named
  after, 221; death of, 219–22; Dredge
  Kang as supervisor, 251; in Japan,
  218; Joël Tan and, 217–22; outreach
  approaches, 130; relationships, 215
Sakakura, Mark, 212–16, 222

Sakakura, Patricia, 212–18, 221–22
San Francisco AIDS Foundation, 72
San Francisco Community Health
  Center, 260
Satrang, 184, 186–90
Schucman, Helen, 155
Schulman, Sarah, 110
Schunhoff, John, 92
Schwartz, Ruth L., 224–25
Search to Involve Pilipino Americans
  (SIPA), 40, 55, 59, 69
segregation in Los Angeles, 5–6,
  72–73
self-esteem approach to prevention,
  121, 131–32
sensitivity training, cross-cultural,
  192–93
Service Network for Asian Pacific
  Youth, 63
7 Steps to Sticky Heaven (Nguyen), 125
sex, 5, 262–63
sex education: abstinence-based, 63;
  harm reduction approach, 124;
  homophobia and, 123; including
  HIV/AIDS in, 63; social marketing
  campaigns, 123–25. *See also*
  safer-sex outreach and
  presentations
sexism. *See* gender and sexism
sexual liberation movement, 17, 21–22
Sexually Compulsives Anonymous
  (SCA), 175
Shanti Foundation, 36, 72, 170–71
Shibata, Kazue, 61, 69
shikata ga nai ("it can't be helped"),
  208–10
Shimabukuro, Wayne, 132, 133*fig.*
Shimada, Margaret Endo, 29–30,
  173–76, 179–82, 210
Siam Media News, 141